OXFORD MEDICAL PUBLICATIONS

KT-431-732

Thyroid disease

THE FACTS

Thyroid Disease

THE FACTS
Second Edition

R. I. S. BAYLISS, KCVO, MD, FRCP
Honorary Consultant Physician and Endocrinologist,
Westminster Hospital, London

and

W. M. G. TUNBRIDGE, MD, FRCP
Consultant Physician,
Newcastle General Hospital, Newcastle upon Tyne

OXFORD NEW YORK TOKYO
OXFORD UNIVERSITY PRESS

Oxford University Press, Walton Street, Oxford OX2 6DP

Oxford New York Toronto
Delhi Bombay Calcutta Madras Karachi
Kuala Lumpur Singapore Hong Kong Tokyo
Nairobi Dar es Salaam Cape Town
Melbourne Auckland Madrid
and associated companies in
Berlin Ibadan

Oxford is a trade mark of Oxford University Press

Published in the United States by
Oxford University Press Inc., New York

First edition 1982
Second edition 1991
Reprinted 1992, 1993

A catalogue record for this book is available from the British Library

Library of Congress Cataloging in Publication Data
Bayliss R. I. S. (Richard Ian Samuel)
Thyroid disease : the facts / R. I. S. Bayliss and W. M. G. Tunbridge.
(Oxford medical publications)
Includes index.
1. Thyroid gland—Diseases. I. Tunbridge, W. M. G. (W. Michael G.)
II. Title. III. Series.
[DNLM: 1. Thyroid Diseases—popular works. WK 200 B358t]
RC655.B39 1991 616.4'4—dc20 91-3227
ISBN 0–19–262104–1 (hbk.)
ISBN 0–19–262103–3 (pbk.)

Printed in Great Britain by
Biddles Ltd
Guildford and King's Lynn

Preface

Why have we written a second edition of this book which is predominantly intended for patients with a thyroid disease and their relatives and friends and for other non-medical readers? The answer is twofold—first, thyroid disorders are common, and second, an understanding of thyroid disorders usually leads to a happier, less worrying, outcome.

How common are thyroid disorders?

The prevalence of thyroid trouble varies considerably in different parts of the world and the incidence is always higher in females than in males. According to the World Health Organization 200 million people world-wide have enlargement of their thyroid gland. Most of these goitres—and 'goitre' simply means enlargement of the thyroid gland—occur in people who live in parts of the world where there is a lack of iodine in the diet, and later we shall see why iodine is so important. However, even in non-deficient iodine areas, enlargement of the thyroid gland, so that it becomes visible, occurs in about 7 per cent of the population and is about ten times more common in women than men. In the United Kingdom some degree of underactivity of the thyroid gland affects about 10 per cent of all women over the age of 45 years. In the United States it is calculated that ten million people have thyroid glands that are either overactive or underactive and in a significant proportion, perhaps as many as two million, this goes unrecognized for many months or years. Thus disorders of the thyroid gland are common, and what is so important is that a significant proportion go unrecognized.

Why should you know about your condition?

Experience has taught us that the more people know about their illnesses, the fewer are their fears. The greater their understanding of what is wrong, the better is their acceptance of, and their co-operation in, the treatment, and the more are they able to help their doctor to help them.
    This is certainly the case in people with disorders of the thyroid gland

who benefit greatly from an understanding of their disease. Notice that in this context we say 'people' rather than 'patients' because many, despite requiring treatment over many years and sometimes indefinitely, may never actually feel ill.

Thus we write mainly for people who have some recognized disorder of the thyroid gland. We write also for their relatives because many thyroid problems or related diseases tend to run in families. If you have a parent, a sister or brother, an aunt or uncle, or a cousin with thyroid disease, you yourself are also more likely to develop, sooner or later, some thyroid disorder. Self-diagnosis is not recommended but, if you are aware of the possibility that you are vulnerable and at risk, the sooner you will seek medical help if you develop any of the symptoms or signs of the diseases described in this book. However, in some instances, disorders of the thyroid gland are insidious in their onset and the changes that occur are so slow to develop that you, and those closest to you, may not be aware of them.

How the thyroid gland works, how it manufactures hormones, and how it is controlled are not hard to understand. We have tried to resist the temptation to be too technical but equally we have done our best not to sacrifice scientific accuracy to over-simplification. In this second edition a glossary is included at the end of the book, where technical terms are explained and more scientific facts are given.

Medicine is not an exact science. It probably never will be, because no two patients are exactly the same. People's susceptibility and their biological and psychological reactions to the same disease will always differ. Equally doctors are likely to vary somewhat in their management of a patient's illness. No one course of action or method of treatment is necessarily more 'right' than another.

You, or your relatives or friends, should not therefore be concerned that the treatment prescribed for you may not always exactly follow the practices advocated in this book. Apparent differences should not upset you because the fundamental scientific principles are widely accepted and likely to be much the same everywhere. Nevertheless, the precise details of management may vary from one centre to another and from one country to another depending upon differences in the population being treated, the availability of technical facilities, laboratory expertise, and, in some instances, financial considerations.

The science of thyroidology is always progressing and, with increased knowledge, changes in the assessment and management of thyroid diseases occur. Hence the need for a second edition of this book.

Nevertheless the art of embracing the special personal needs and wishes, the environmental or social factors, and the idiosyncrasies of an individual patient with a thyroid disorder may contribute as much to the successful outcome as the science does.

This book owes much to our colleagues in this country and abroad, particularly in the United States. It is, however, the patients from many lands, whom we have treated or supervised, who have undoubtedly taught us the most. To them go our special thanks.

Finally a word to the patient who, having recently been diagnosed as having some thyroid disorder, is reading this book for the first time. We suggest you start by reading the chapter relevant to your condition. For example, if you have an overactive thyroid gland due to Graves' disease read Chapter 4, or if you have an underactive gland due to Hashimoto's auto-immune thyroiditis first read Chapter 7. You may find that you have other symptoms you have not mentioned to your doctor or not previously recognized yourself. This you may find reassuring. Then go back to the beginning of the book and read Chapters 1 and 2. This will help to orientate you. Then read Chapter 3 about the tests and the investigations that have been, or will be, done to confirm the diagnosis of your illness. This will help you to co-operate in your treatment and later to assess your own improvement.

We are grateful to Mr Keith Duguid, formerly Head of the Department of Medical Illustration at Westminster Hospital, for the photographic work and to Dr C.R. Bayliss, Consultant Radiologist at the Royal Devon and Exeter Hospital, for the illustrations used in Plate 4. Dr Robert H. Phillips, Consultant Radiotherapist and Oncologist at Westminster Hospital, London, kindly gave advice about the use of radioactive isotopes.

London   R.I.S.B.
Newcastle upon Tyne   W.M.G.T.
1991

Contents

At the end of each chapter are answers to some of the more common questions which are asked about thyroid disease.

1

The thyroid gland

Where is the thyroid gland?

Normally the thyroid gland lies in the front of your neck just below your Adam's apple in the position where the knot of a man's tie would be (Fig. 1). The gland is H-shaped and consists of two lobes joined together in the middle. The left and right lobes, each about the size and shape of half a plum cut vertically, lie on either side of the mid-line against the windpipe, and are connected by a bridge of thyroid tissue, known as the isthmus, which runs across the front of the windpipe (Fig. 1).

In men a normal thyroid gland is seldom sufficiently large to be visible, but in a young woman with a thin neck it may just be discernible, particularly when the chin is lifted up. If visible the gland will be seen to move up and down as you swallow. In young people with a thin neck your doctor may be able to feel the two lobes of the thyroid but in older

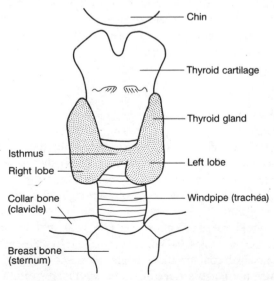

Fig. 1 The anatomy of the thyroid gland.

people with a short or thick neck it may not be palpable. A healthy gland is smooth and is not tender. It is not lumpy or hard.

In some perfectly normal people the gland may extend downwards to lie wholly or partially behind the upper part of the breast-bone or sternum. This is called a retrosternal thyroid.

Where does the thyroid come from?

In the baby developing in the womb (the fetus) the thyroid gland has its origins at the root of the tongue. As the fetus grows the thyroid moves down the neck and long before the baby is born it occupies the usual adult position. The path of this descent is marked by a narrow cord, the thyroglossal duct, running from the tongue (the glossus) to the neck. The bottom inch or two of this duct may contain thyroid tissue and is then called the pyramidal lobe. This extra lobe of the thyroid extends upwards from the isthmus and may lie in the mid-line or on either side of the larynx.

What happens if the thyroid does not descend properly?

Very rarely in some babies the thyroid gland does not descend properly and remains in its original position near the root of the tongue. A mis-placed thyroid gland like this seldom functions properly, and is an important but uncommon cause of deficient thyroid hormone production in new-born babies (Chapter 8).

What does the thyroid do?

The thyroid manufactures certain chemical substances (hormones) that are passed into the bloodstream and act on cells and tissues elsewhere in your body. Other glands like the thyroid that produce hormones include the pituitary, the ovary and the testis, among others, and are known as endocrine glands.

The thyroid makes two hormones. One is thyroxine which, because it contains four atoms of iodine, is also called T_4. The other is triiodo-thyronine which contains three iodine atoms and for brevity is called T_3. Both these hormones are secreted into the bloodstream and are carried round the body. In the distant tissues the thyroxine is converted to triiodothyronine and it is the triiodothyronine that actually influences the distant cells.

What do the thyroid hormones do?

The thyroid hormones control the speed of activity of all body cells. Too little of the thyroid hormones means that the body cells work at too slow a rate; too much causes them to work too fast.

The action of the thyroid hormones is in many respects like the speed control on your record player. If a 45 r.p.m. disc is played with the speed control set at 33⅓ r.p.m. the music is slow and lugubrious. This is the equivalent to thyroid deficiency or hypothyroidism. If a 33⅓ r.p.m. disc is played with the speed control set at 45 r.p.m. the music is squeaky, hurried and has a 'Mickey Mouse' sound. This is like overactivity of the thyroid gland when too much thyroid hormone is secreted and the cells of the body work faster than is normal.

Although the two thyroid hormones have a similar effect and influence the proper working of all body cells, their action is particularly evident in certain tissues and for certain functions. For example the growth and development, both physical and mental, of a baby depend upon the presence of the correct amount of the thyroid hormones. We also see this in the animal world. Without thyroxine a tadpole will not change into a frog, and without thyroxine in the correct amount a new-born baby will not grow properly nor will its brain develop properly. Similarly, in a child, too little thyroid hormone will slow-up growth, whereas too much may make the child grow faster than normal. Thyroid hormones have a very noticeable effect, as we shall see later, on the heart and the heart rate in particular.

Fundamentally the thyroid hormones regulate the rate of oxygen consumption, which is another way of saying they control the speed of activity of the body cells. This metabolic action influences the utilization of the main components in our food—sugars, proteins, and fats. When there is thyroid deficiency, for example, the level of a particular fat, cholesterol, usually increases in the bloodstream. If this is allowed to continue the arteries may become furred up because the cholesterol is deposited in the inner wall of the blood-vessels which become narrowed.

The manufacture of thyroid hormones

Thyroxine and triiodothyronine are formed in the cells of the thyroid gland. Both hormones contain iodine, and thus iodine is essential for their manufacture or synthesis. This essential raw material is extracted from the bloodstream by the specialized thyroid cells. Inside the cells of the thyroid gland, the iodine is amalgamated with other substances in a number of chemical steps to form T_4 and T_3. Once formed the two hormones are stored in parking areas within the gland. The 'parked' hormones are released from storage into the bloodstream as and when the body cells need them.

Where does the iodine come from?

Normally iodine is provided by the food we eat, particularly fish. Iodine also comes from the soil, in which our crops grow to provide us with bread and vegetables, and on which cows graze to give us milk. The iodine is derived from the rain that falls on the soil, and this in turn comes from the water vapourized from the sea to form the rain. In parts of the world far removed from the sea the soil is likely to be deficient in iodine. This happens in the land round the Congo in Central Africa, in the Andes in South America, the Himalayas in the Indian subcontinent, Switzerland in Central Europe, around the Great Lakes in the USA and in certain areas in other land masses such as Spain and Iran. People living in these areas may have difficulty in making thyroid hormones because there is insufficient iodine in their diet. Hence public-health measures have to be taken to supplement their dietary intake of iodine.

How is the secretion of thyroid hormones controlled?

What determines the amount of thyroid hormones secreted into the bloodstream? There is a clever mechanism for this which is simple to understand. Fundamentally it works like the control of the central heating in your home. The thermostat in your hall or living room senses the temperature. If the temperature falls below a certain pre-set level, the thermostat activates the oil-fired or gas furnace to produce more heat. When the temperature rises to or above the pre-set level, the thermostat turns the furnace off or reduces its heat production.

Look upon the thyroid gland as the furnace and the pituitary gland— or certain cells in it—as the thermostat. The pituitary gland is the size of a grape and lies at the base of your brain. It has been called the conductor of the endocrine orchestra, and it secretes many different hormones that regulate the other endocrine glands. The hormone we are interested in now is the thyroid-stimulating hormone, also known as TSH or thyro-trophin. TSH passes into the bloodstream and activates the thyroid gland to release the stored thyroid hormones, to manufacture more of them, and to extract more iodine from the blood to do so. As a result of this stimulation of the thyroid cells, the level of the thyroid hormones in the bloodstream rises. The cells in the pituitary that secrete TSH sense this, just as your thermostat senses the rise in the temperature in your sitting room. When the level of the thyroid hormones reaches a certain point, the secretion of TSH by the pituitary is reduced and the furnace (the thyroid gland) stops working so hard. This is what is called a feed-back control mechanism (Fig. 2).

The pituitary gland is very sensitive to the levels of the thyroid hormones circulating in the blood. It is also responsive to other signals

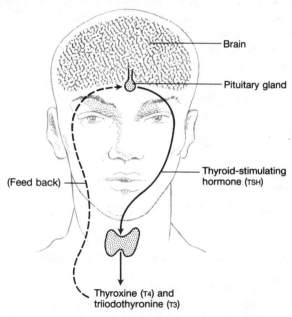

Brain

Pituitary gland

Thyroid-stimulating hormone (TSH)

(Feed back)

Thyroxine (T4) and triiodothyronine (T3)

Fig. 2 Mechanism controlling the secretion by the thyroid gland of thyroxine (T_4) and triiodothyronine (T_3). As the levels of T_4 and T_3 rise in the blood-stream, the secretion of the thyroid-stimulating hormone (TSH) from the pituitary gland is reduced or switched off (feedback control mechanism). As the levels of T_4 and T_3 fall, the pituitary gland secretes more TSH so that activity of the thyroid gland is increased.

from higher in the brain, particularly from another little gland called the hypothalamus.

How do the thyroid hormones get around in the bloodstream?

The answer is that both hormones are mainly carried loosely attached to certain proteins in the blood. In a sense you can look upon the hormones as coal being carried in an open coal truck (the hormone-carrying proteins). More than 99.9 per cent of the two hormones are transported in this way. However, while attached to these carrier proteins the hormones are biologically inactive, just as you cannot use the coal in a coal truck unless you first take it out of the truck. Only when the thyroid hormones are freed from their protein-binding do they become biologically active at the cellular level. Some of the hormones, less than a fraction of 1 per cent of the total, are not attached to the carrier proteins and are floating free, as it were, in the water of your blood. This unattached hormone is biologically active.

You will hear a little more about this later because the protein-bound and the so-called free hormones are important when it comes to measuring the levels of T_4 and T_3 in the blood. Sometimes changes occur in the carrier-proteins so that more, or less, of the hormone is protein-bound with less, or more, of the hormone being free, unbound and biologically active.

Questions and Answers

$Q.1$ What is the thyroid gland?

$A.$ It is a small endocrine gland that controls the activity of your body cells.

$Q.2$ Where is the thyroid gland?

$A.$ It lies in the front of your neck in the position where a man knots his tie.

$Q.3$ What does the thyroid do?

$A.$ It produces the thyroid hormones which are chemical messengers sent to the rest of the body.

*Q.*4   What controls the output of thyroid hormones?

A.   The output depends upon the level of thyroid hormones in your blood. If the level falls, the pituitary gland releases more thyroid-stimulating hormone (TSH) which stimulates the gland to produce more hormones and release them into the bloodstream.

2

Things that go wrong with the thyroid

Certain conditions afflict only the thyroid gland and do not, indeed cannot, occur elsewhere in any other tissue or organ in your body. For example, overactivity of the thyroid (hyperthyroidism) in which too much hormone is secreted, and underactivity (hypothyroidism) in which too little hormone is secreted, are disorders peculiar and specific to the thyroid and produce characteristic symptoms. On the other hand certain other disorders of the thyroid gland such as infections, inflammation, and cancer, are not so unique to the thyroid because similar changes may occur in other organs. Nevertheless the symptoms and the clinical picture induced by infection, inflammation, or cancer are strongly coloured by the fact that the disease process is located in the thyroid.

Let us take a brief preliminary look at some of the common disorders that may affect the thyroid.

Increase in size

Enlargement of the thyroid gland from any cause is called a goitre. The whole gland may be enlarged uniformly or only one part of it. A goitre may vary in size from a thyroid gland that feels slightly larger than normal, to one that is clearly visible (Fig. 3a), and on to one that is a large lump the size of a small melon (Fig. 3b).

Many disorders of the thyroid gland cause it to become enlarged. The enlargement may be associated with a normal output of thyroid hormones, and the patient is then said to be euthyroid. The goitre may be associated with an increased secretion of thyroid hormone, and the patient is then said to be hyperthyroid. Or it may be associated with a deficient output and the patient is then hypothyroid. From this you will see that the size of the thyroid gland bears little relationship to its secretory activity. A small goitre or even a thyroid gland of normal size

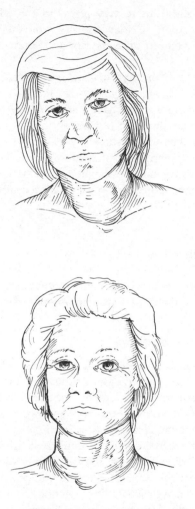

Fig. 3   (a) A medium-sized goitre. (b) A large nodular goitre in a patient living
in an iodine-deficient area of the world.

may produce excess thyroid hormones, whereas a large goitre may be
associated with deficient secretion.

Goitres are usually painless but in some conditions the gland hurts and
is tender on pressure. If sufficiently large the goitre may cause some
discomfort on swallowing. If a goitre becomes very large it is not only

cosmetically unsightly but it may press on the windpipe and cause difficulty with breathing. It may also press on the veins in the neck carrying blood to the heart from the face and brain and cause a sense of fullness in the head.

Slight enlargement of the thyroid gland is so common in women at the time of puberty and during pregnancy that it is looked upon as normal. Do not be self-conscious if you have a small goitre, which seldom is as unsightly as you may think. In fact not so long ago a small goitre was considered a mark of beauty, as shown by many of the portraits of elegant women painted by the prolific Dutch court painter Lely (1619–1680).

The cause of a goitre must be sought and the necessary steps taken to stop it from becoming larger. A more detailed account of goitres is given in Chapters 10 and 11.

Auto-immune disorders

The thyroid gland is particularly prone to auto-immune disorders, but first we must explain what an auto-immune disorder is.

What is an auto-immune disorder?

All of us have an immune system which protects us from infection with commonly encountered bacteria and viruses. A baby inherits some of its immunity from its mother, particularly if the baby is breast-fed. Later in life the baby meets these infections and develops what is usually a life-long immunity to them. How does this immune system work?

In the blood are certain white corpuscle cells called lymphocytes which are on the look-out for the 'foreign' proteins that occur in micro-organisms and viruses—'foreign' because the proteins are not a constituent of the normal individual. The lymphocytes spot that the proteins are 'foreign' and develop chemical substances called antibodies that neutralize them. The situation is like soldiers becoming aware that foreign enemy troops have penetrated their defences. Just as the soldiers round up the enemy troops to disarm or kill them, so the lymphocytes react by producing antibodies that neutralize or kill the invading micro-organisms comprised of 'foreign' proteins.

Foreign proteins of any sort are looked upon as invading enemies and antibodies are formed against them. This is why there are problems when a tissue like skin or an organ like a kidney or a heart, essentially made of protein, is transplanted from one person to another. The lymphocytes of the recipient of the transplant look upon the donated tissue or organ as 'foreign', which it is. The white cells form antibodies which attack the transplant and, without special intervention by the doctor, would destroy it. This rejection by the recipient is one of the major problems in transplant surgery.

In auto-immune disorders, for reasons we do not yet fully understand, the lymphocytes get the idea that some tissue or organ in your body does not belong to you; it should not be there; it is 'foreign'. Antibodies are produced that mount an attack on the 'self' in the mistaken belief that the tissue is 'foreign'. It is like a group of soldiers suddenly getting the idea that the troops serving alongside them in the same regiment belong to the enemy.

In the case of auto-immune thyroid disorders, the lymphocytes produce antibodies that react with the cells, or certain constituents of the cells, of the thyroid gland. The presence and strength of these antibodies can be measured in your blood.

Some antibodies are destructive and kill off the thyroid cells. Other antibodies stimulate the thyroid cells to produce too much thyroid hormone. Occasionally destructive and stimulating antibodies occur together and usually after having an overactive thyroid gland for a time the patient becomes thyroid deficient.

Hyperthyroidism

An increase above the normal level of thyroxine or triiodothyronine or both causes thyroid overactivity (hyperthyroidism or thyrotoxicosis). The commonest cause of this is an auto-immune disease called Graves' disease, named after the Dublin physician, Dr Robert Graves, who described the condition in three young women in 1835. In the English-speaking world auto-immune hyperthyroidism still bears his name. In Europe, however, Graves' disease is known as Basedow's disease after Carl von Basedow who, in 1840, published a very clear account of the condition which so often is characterized by a goitre, palpitations of the heart and changes in the eyes.

In hyperthyroidism, or thyrotoxicosis as it is also called, the metabolism of the cells in the body is increased. The turntable on the record player is turning round too fast (p. 3). The clinical picture varies some-what depending upon your age but the commonest features are a rapid heart rate, palpitations and cardiac consciousness, a rapid bowel rate causing loose motions or diarrhoea, and an increased metabolism causing loss of weight. Graves' disease, in which antibodies stimulate the thyroid cells to secrete excess thyroid hormones, is considered in Chapter 4. The commonly associated eye changes are discussed in Chapter 5. Other less common causes of hyperthyroidism are dealt with in Chapter 6.

Hypothyroidism

Underactivity of the thyroid gland may have many different causes and is discussed in Chapters 7 and 8. World-wide iodine deficiency is the commonest cause of thyroid deficiency at any age, but in the Western World the commonest cause of hypothyroidism is chronic auto-immune thyroiditis, also known as lymphadenoid or chronic lymphocytic goitre, or Hashimoto's disease after the Japanese surgeon who described the appearance of the gland in 1912 (Chapter 7).

In hypothyroidism the body cells work sluggishly. The turntable of the record player is turning round too slowly (p. 3). The heart rate slows, the bowels are sluggish leading to constipation, the skin becomes dry and thickened, the voice is deeper and croaky and you become intolerant of cold. The clinical features are discussed in detail in Chapter 8.

Thyroiditis

Infection and inflammation of the thyroid gland are not uncommon. The most common cause of this thyroid inflammation is a virus. This subacute viral thyroiditis, also called de Quervain's thyroiditis after a Swiss physician who first described it, is 'subacute' because the degree of discomfort in the neck due to inflammation of the thyroid gland is usually not very severe but it tends to persist for several weeks or months if left untreated. The gland hurts and is tender to the touch; swallowing may be painful.

The inflammation may temporarily cause excess amounts of thyroid hormones to leach out of the gland and for some weeks you will suffer from thyroid overactivity (thyrotoxicosis). Sometimes the virus infection causes no discomfort at all in the thyroid gland, and the associated hyperthyroidism is then attributed to 'silent thyroiditis' (p. 107). Subacute viral thyroiditis is discussed in Chapter 9.

Very rarely the thyroid is infected by bacterial micro-organisms such as the common streptococcus that may cause an associated acute sore throat, a staphylococcus that commonly causes boils (furunculosis), or the tubercle bacillus (p. 110).

Cancer

Among disorders of the thyroid gland cancer is rare, and among malignant growths in the body as a whole it is even rarer. Most thyroid cancers are well differentiated; this means that the cells that make up the cancer continue to look like relatively normal thyroid cells under the microscope. These malignant cells do not usually multiply rapidly and hence the tumour does not grow fast. Not only do the cancer cells look rather like normal thyroid cells but they often behave like them. For instance, they usually remain responsive to the action of thyroid-stimulating hormone and they continue to extract iodine from the bloodstream. This means that in addition to surgical removal of the growth, which is the usual initial treatment, any remaining malignant cells can be eliminated by treatment with radioactive iodine (Chapter 12).

Provided the condition is diagnosed early, the treatment of a differentiated thyroid cancer is usually very successful.

Questions and Answers

Q.1   If I develop a goitre, does it mean I've got cancer?

A.   Certainly not. Thyroid cancer is very rare and there are a great many more common non-malignant conditions that cause enlargement of the thyroid.

Q.2   What is an auto-immune disease?

A.   It is a disorder of your immune system, which gets the mistaken idea that some organ or tissue in your body does not belong to you, but is 'foreign' and should be got rid of.

Q.3   In an auto-immune disease how does my body try to get rid of the allegedly 'foreign' cells?

A.   Certain chemicals, auto-antibodies, are developed that attack the supposedly 'foreign' cells.

Q.4   Are the auto-antibodies always destructive?

A.   No, sometimes they can stimulate your thyroid gland to increased secretory activity as happens in Graves' disease.

3

How the doctor finds out what is wrong

To find out what is wrong with your thyroid gland, your doctor will first wish to hear all about your symptoms. Do tell your doctor everything. Do not omit any symptom just because *you* think it is irrelevant; it may not be. After listening to you, the doctor will probably need to ask you a number of questions either for you to expand on certain things you have found wrong with yourself or to discuss matters that you have not mentioned.

Then you will be examined. In addition to the general physical examination particular attention will be given to your weight (and height in the case of children), your pulse rate, and the findings in your neck. The doctor may measure the circumference of your neck.

If you have any eye symptoms the distance between the front of each eye and the edge of the bony socket in which the eye lies may be painlessly measured in clinics that specialize in thyroid disorders (Fig. 5; p. 48). Additional eye tests may be arranged and photographs taken of your neck and of your eyes.

Almost certainly blood and other tests will be carried out. These can be divided into two main groups.

1. Tests to tell whether your thyroid is putting out the correct amount, or too little or too much, of the thyroid hormones;

2. Tests designed to give information as to what is wrong with your thyroid gland. These will help to answer such questions as:
   - Why is my thyroid gland enlarged?
   - Why is my gland overactive (or underactive)?
   - Why have I got a lump in my thyroid; is it serious?
   - Why is the front of my neck so sore?

Direct tests of thyroid function

Over the years many different methods have been used to determine
whether your thyroid gland is making the right amount of thyroid
hormones. Modern tests are carried out on a small sample of blood taken
from a vein, and usually the results are available quite quickly.
Regrettably it must, however, be admitted that no one single test of
thyroid function is always one hundred per cent diagnostically reliable
because a result that is too high or too low may occur for a number of
different reasons (see Glossary, pp. 125 and 126).

Thyroid-stimulating hormone (TSH) level

With modern techniques, normal, high, and low levels of TSH can be
measured accurately. Of course the level of TSH is not exactly the same
in every healthy person, and the normal or reference range is that which
is found in 95 per cent of healthy people. This range will vary from one
laboratory to another depending on the exact technical procedure used
and the normal population being studied by that laboratory.

The underactive gland.   In hypothyroidism when the secretion of
thyroid hormones is reduced, the pituitary gland responds by secreting
more TSH in order to increase the activity of the flagging thyroid. The
TSH level is increased roughly in proportion to the decrease in the
thyroxine level. Thus in established hypothyroidism with all the characteristic clinical symptoms and signs, the TSH level is very high. When
the degree of thyroid underactivity is more marginal, before any florid
evidence of it may have appeared and the thyroxine level is at or just
below its lower normal range, the TSH will be increased to a lesser
degree, but this is of great help in confirming that the thyroid gland is
having to struggle. Indeed, experience has shown that, in the diagnosis of
the failing thyroid, the TSH level is the most sensitive test for detecting
this.

The overactive gland.   When the thyroid is overactive and increased
amounts of thyroid hormones are being secreted, the pituitary gland is
switched off by the feed-back mechanism (p. 4 and Fig. 2). The TSH
level falls below normal. This test is therefore of value in helping to
confirm a diagnosis of hyperthyroidism when the TSH will be below the

bottom of the reference range and may even be undetectable. However, low levels of TSH may also occur in circumstances other than hyperthyroidism (see Glossary, p. 125).

Serum thyroxine (T_4) level

Both the total amount of thyroxine in the bloodstream, which is largely bound to carrier-proteins, or the free thyroxine which is the tiny amount floating free in the water of your blood can be measured. Some laboratories measure the total T_4 and others the free T_4. The advantages and disadvantages of the two methods are discussed in the Glossary (p. 126).

Hyperthyroidism.   Raised levels of thyroxine occur in most cases of hyperthyroidism but sometimes only the level of triiodothyronine (T_3) is raised. The more severe the overactivity of the gland the higher are the blood hormone levels.

Hypothyroidism.   Reduced levels of thyroxine occur in most cases of hypothyroidism but not always to a marked degree in the early stages (see Chapter 8).

The main trouble with measuring the total thyroxine compared with the free thyroxine level is that the former is influenced so much by the level of the carrier-proteins to which the T_4 is loosely attached, and may not truly reflect your thyroid status. Sometimes an additional test is used to make allowance for variations in the proteins that carry thyroxine in the bloodstream. This test is known as the T_3-resin binding test (p. 127) and from the result the free thyroxine index can be calculated (see below).

Free thyroxine index

The free thyroxine index reflects that amount of thyroxine which is unattached to protein and is free in the blood in much the same way as the free thyroxine test does. It is the unbound thyroxine that we really want to know about because the free thyroxine determines your thyroid status. It is for this reason that in many centres measurement of the free thyroxine test is now used in preference to the total serum thyroxine, the T_3-resin binding, and the free thyroxine index tests.

Serum triiodothyronine (T_3) level

Both the total (protein-bound) and the free T_3 levels can be measured. High levels occur if you have an overactive thyroid. In some patients with hyperthyroidism the T_3 level rises, some weeks or months, earlier than the thyroxine level does. Indeed there are some patients with thyrotoxicosis with a raised T_3 level who never develop a raised thyroxine level. Thus if you have symptoms and signs suggestive of hyperthyroidism and a low TSH level but a normal level of thyroxine, the finding of a high T_3 (total or free) will explain the situation which is known as T_3-toxicosis.

The T_3 level is less useful in the diagnosis of hypothyroidism because the failing thyroid gland finds it easier to produce triiodothyronine than thyroxine. Thus the level of T_3 falls later and more slowly than the thyroxine does.

Low levels of T_3 may also occur in patients suffering from many physical and psychiatric illnesses quite unrelated to the thyroid gland. This is called the 'sick euthyroid' syndrome and the T_3 level gradually returns to normal as the patient recovers (p. 109).

Combined tests

A great deal can be said for assessing the secretory activity of the thyroid from two different angles by doing two different *types* of thyroid function tests:

- the level of the thyroid hormones on the one hand; and
- the secretion of TSH on the other.

Except when the diagnosis is obvious, your doctor is likely to assess the situation by measuring *either* the total or free T_4 (and in suspected hyperthyroidism the total or free T_3) *and* the TSH level if you are suspected of having overactivity or underactivity of the thyroid gland.

Table 1 summarizes some of the results that may be obtained by measuring the free thyroxine, the free triiodothyronine, and the TSH levels.

Indirect tests of thyroid function

A number of indirect tests may be used to assess thyroid secretory function.

Table 1   A summary of some common results of tests of thyroid
secretory function and their significance

Free T_4 level	Free T_3 level	TSH level	Significance
High	High	Low	Hyperthyroidism or excess treatment with T_4
Normal	High	Low	T_3-Toxicosis
Normal	Normal	Normal	Normal euthyroid
Normal or high	Normal	Normal	Euthyroid on treatment with T_4
Normal or low	Low	Normal or low	Generalized ill-health; 'sick euthyroid' syndrome
Low or normal	Normal	High	Subclinical or mild hypothyroidism
Low	Low or normal	High	Hypothyroidism

Radio-iodine uptake

This test is based upon the uptake by the thyroid gland of one of the
radioactive isotopes of iodine. In hyperthyroidism the production of
excess thyroid hormones requires more of the essential raw material,
namely iodine. Hence the thyroid has to take more iodine out of the
bloodstream for hormone synthesis. Conversely in hypothyroidism less
iodine, or radioactive iodine, is trapped because less than normal
amounts of thyroid hormones are being made.

The uptake of radio-iodine is measured by you taking by mouth, or
being given by injection, a radioactive isotope. The radioactivity in your
thyroid is measured with a counter placed over your neck after 2–6 hours
if you are suspected of having an overactive gland and after 24–48 hours
if you are suspected of having an underactive one.

This is an indirect method of assessing the production of thyroid hormones. The situation is similar to that in a motorcar factory in which
iodine is akin to the steel going into the plant. It can be argued that the
more raw material (in this case steel) that goes into the factory the more
cars are coming out the other end. Over a prolonged period of time this
would probably be true, but in the short term all sorts of fallacies may

arise. The factory might be stockpiling steel and holding it in store without increasing car production. The factory might be making the usual number of cars but storing them in the plant and not releasing them for distribution. Similarly with iodine, an increase in uptake may indicate stockpiling, perhaps because the thyroid gland has been, for a time, starved of iodine. Thus increased uptake cannot invariably be equated with increased production of thyroid hormones. Even though the thyroid may be capable of normal hormone synthesis, the uptake of iodine will be suppressed if you are taking T_4 or T_3 by mouth because such medication will depress the secretion of TSH by the pituitary and the thyroid will be in an inactive resting state.

One of the most instructive examples of a possibly misleading result being obtained by measuring the uptake of radio-iodine to assess thyroid secretory function is in subacute viral thyroiditis (Chapter 9). In this condition the thyroid cells are disorganised by the inflammation caused by the virus. They cannot work properly and hence the uptake of iodine is zero. However the inflammatory process causes preformed thyroid hormones stored in the gland to be released into the circulation so that the symptoms and signs of hyperthyroidism develop.

Various slightly different isotopes of iodine are used, often a tracer amount of ^{131}I but sometimes ^{123}I or ^{132}I because they have a shorter radioactive life than ^{131}I and they decay more quickly, hence causing less irradiation to your body in general. They are preferred for studies in children and whenever repeated tests are made. If you are given these isotopes in trace amounts you can confidently be reassured that the irradiation hazard is negligible but even so they will not be used if you are pregnant because the radioisotope will enter the thyroid gland of your baby.

Nowadays for reasons of convenience another isotope called technetium (^{99m}Tc) is often used in place of iodine isotopes. This is taken up by the thyroid cells in the same way as iodine is trapped but it is not incorporated in the making of the thyroid hormones. Technetium and the iodine isotopes now find their main use in determining what is wrong with the thyroid gland (p. 23) rather than in assessing its secretory function.

Ankle-reflex time

The speed of tendon reflexes, such as the well-known reaction when the tendon just below your knee-cap is tapped with a hammer, is influenced by the level of thyroid hormones. In practice the ankle reflex, judged by tapping on the Achilles tendon at the back of your heel, is the one used and the speed of the movement of your foot may be recorded with an electronic device. The reflex time is often much slowed in hypothyroidism and is quicker than normal in hyperthyroidism. This test is influenced by factors other than the circulating levels of the thyroid hormones. Although it can be useful in assessing your response to treatment, it is of limited value in the primary assessment of thyroid function.

Cholesterol

The level of cholesterol, a particular type of fat in the blood, is influenced by the amount of thyroid hormones secreted. In hypothyroidism the cholesterol is usually substantially raised above normal and in hyperthyroidism it is often low. However the cholesterol is influenced by many other factors. Variations from normal in thyroid disease may occur only when the degree of disordered secretory function is extreme and of long standing.

Tests to determine the cause of thyroid disease

Having assessed whether your thyroid is functioning normally or not, your doctor will need to find out what exactly has gone wrong. For instance you may have a goitre but thyroid secretory function is normal. Why then have you developed a goitre? Equally if your gland is under-active or overactive, your doctor must find out why.

It is not enough to decide that you are, for example, hypothyroid by finding that the free thyroxine level is low and the TSH level is high. The next question to be asked and answered is 'what has gone wrong with this thyroid gland to make it underactive?' This may be obvious if you have been previously treated for hyperthyroidism with radio-iodine or by surgery. In less obvious cases there are many possible reasons, such as iodine deficiency or more probably Hashimoto's disease.

Investigations may help to decide if a lump in the thyroid is a hollow cyst or a solid nodule, and whether it is benign (non-cancerous) or malignant (Chapters 11 and 12).

It is also necessary to determine whether hyperthyroidism is due to an auto-immune process that induces the whole gland to secrete excess thyroid hormones (Graves' disease) or to temporary thyroiditis, or whether it is due to a localized area of overactive cells producing too much hormone (a toxic adenoma). These distinctions are important because they have a significant bearing on the best treatment for you.

Hence the investigations discussed in this section are directed at finding out why the thyroid is behaving abnormally. Not all these tests are likely to be required and the order in which they are done will vary according to what your doctor suspects has gone wrong.

Thyroid antibodies

As explained on page 10 in Chapter 2 antibodies may develop in your body which act on the cells of the thyroid gland in different ways. Detection of these antibodies and assessment of their level may be crucial in deciding what is wrong with you.

Thyroid-inhibiting antibodies. A variety of antibodies may impair thyroid function but the most important of these is the microsomal antibody. This is cytotoxic which means that it destroys thyroid cells. It is usually found in the blood of patients with Hashimoto's disease and is directly responsible for the gradual destruction of the thyroid with the subsequent development of hypothyroidism. This auto-immune destruction is a slow process and takes place over many months or years. At the present time we do not have a safe and effective way of arresting the destructive process, but the knowledge that this antibody is present will ensure that a careful eye is kept on you so that replacement therapy with thyroxine is given as soon as, or even before, the thyroid ceases to secrete an adequate amount of hormones.

It is also important to know that you have an auto-immune disorder of the thyroid gland because this is sometimes, but rarely, associated sooner or later with other auto-immune diseases (Chapter 15). Thus your doctor may wish, for example, to check for the presence of an antibody that destroys certain cells in the stomach, the secretion of which is responsible for the absorption of vitamin B_{12}—a vitamin essential for the making of the red corpuscles in your blood. If this antibody is found to be present, a check must be kept on your haemoglobin level and at the earliest evidence of anaemia developing injections of vitamin B_{12} given (p. 112).

Thyroid-stimulating antibodies. Antibodies that increase thyroid activity are the probable cause of Graves' disease. These thyroid-stimulating substances can be detected in about 90 per cent of patients with Graves' disease and occur also in 60 per cent of patients who have the eye complications of Graves' disease but are not thyrotoxic (Chapter 5). The same antibodies may occur in those patients with Hashimoto's disease who have a transient episode of hyperthyroidism ('Hashitoxicosis', p. 59).

Radioisotope thyroid scan

In this investigation you are given a radioisotope, either technetium or iodine, that is taken up by your thyroid gland. Temporarily the gland becomes radioactive and this is charted by a counter placed over your neck. The amount of radioactive material to which you are exposed is very small and you need have no fears as to the amount of irradiation your body receives. A record of the uptake in your neck (the scintigram) may be charted on X-ray film or on paper in colour as shown in Plate 1 (reproduced here in black and white).

A normal thyroid isotope scan will show that the gland is located in the right place. It will show the right and left lobes to be of approximately equal size. It may not always show the isthmus.

The uptake of the isotope is uniform throughout both lobes but the radioactivity is greater in the centre of each lobe than at the edges because there is more thyroid tissue in the middle of the lobe.

If the thyroid gland does not develop properly or its descent into the neck from its origins at the base of the tongue is abnormal (see Chapter 1), the scintigram will show little radioactivity and this may be located high in the neck under the chin. These findings are mainly of importance when seeking the cause of hypothyroidism in a baby or a child.

When the thyroid descends too far, the scan will usually show some activity in the lower part of the neck but most of the activity is found behind the upper part of the breastbone (a retrosternal thyroid) or more rarely lower down in the chest (a mediastinal thyroid).

Hyperthyroidism. When there is overactivity of the thyroid the scan may show one of four different appearances depending upon the cause.

- In Graves' disease the whole gland is overactive, and the scan shows high activity uniformly throughout both lobes. The lobes are usually, but not always, enlarged.
- When the thyrotoxicosis is caused by overactivity in just one clump of cells (a toxic adenoma), the radioactivity is almost totally confined

to this area of hyperactivity (Plate 2). This is referred to as a 'hot' nodule because of the excess uptake of isotope in this one area. The rest of the gland takes up little or no isotope and is 'cold' because it is inactive as a result of the excess thyroid hormones formed by the hot nodule depressing the pituitary secretion of TSH through the normal feedback mechanism.

- In a multinodular toxic goitre the isotope uptake is largely confined to a number of different areas which vary in size and in their 'hotness'. Thus the scan shows multiple 'warm' nodules separated by areas of inactive 'cold' tissue.

- When hyperthyroidism is caused by viral thyroiditis, the working of the thyroid gland is so disrupted that it temporarily ceases to function and the scan shows very little or no uptake. The thyrotoxicosis is due to preformed thyroid hormones being discharged from the inflamed gland. With recovery from the inflammation, the gland will show a normal uptake again some months after the initial illness.

Because the treatment of these different causes of hyperthyroidism is not the same, it is important that the distinction is made. Of course an isotope scan is not necessary in every hyperthyroid patient because the diagnosis may be obvious if you have thyrotoxicosis together with the eye signs of Graves' ophthalmopathy. In some cases of viral thyroiditis the diagnosis is also obvious to your doctor from your history of a 'flu-like illness followed by pain and tenderness in the thyroid and the symptoms and signs of thyrotoxicosis. However some cases of thyroiditis are not associated with an obvious 'flu-like illness and the thyroid gland is not painful (so-called 'silent thyroiditis', p. 107).

Nodular or lumpy goitres. Isotope scans are helpful in deciding the nature of a lump or lumps in one or both lobes of your thyroid gland. Quite often we see a patient who has noticed a lump in her neck, which may be completely painless and perhaps the size of a grape. On examination the lump is found to be part of the thyroid gland: on swallowing it moves with the rest of the gland which feels perfectly normal. A scan with ^{131}I or ^{123}I may show that the nodule does not take up the isotope and is 'cold' (Plate 3). This makes it slightly more likely that the nodule could be malignant but in fact most, about 80 per cent, 'cold' nodules when biopsied (see below) or removed for examination under the microscope prove not to be malignant. Sometimes an isotope scan carried out to investigate what appears on examination to be a solitary nodule shows that not only is the nodule 'cold' but that there are other 'cold' areas in the rest of the gland which your doctor cannot feel. This is helpful because it shows that you have multiple 'cold' nodules, not a solitary one, and this makes it even less likely that malignant change has occurred.

Thus isotope scanning with radio-iodine is useful in the assessment of patients with thyroid lumps (Chapter 11) and invaluable in the management of those with thyroid cancer (Chapter 12).

Ultrasound scan

This technique, also sometimes called a sonogram or echogram, is painless. Some jelly is spread over your neck and a probe moved backwards and forwards across your thyroid gland. This probe sends an inaudible painless 'sound' wave through the skin and into your thyroid gland which is then reflected back to a receiver in the probe.

As the probe is moved from side to side a pattern emerges (Plate 4), just as when this technique is used for locating a submarine or a wreck on the seabed. The ultrasound will show the size of your thyroid gland, whether a lump is a solid nodule or a hollow cyst filled with fluid and whether there is a single nodule or several.

Biopsy

A biopsy is removal of a small piece of thyroid tissue for examination under the microscope. This is helpful because a careful study of a piece of tissue can often tell your doctor what exactly is wrong; for example whether a nodule is benign or malignant. A fine needle biopsy is a virtually painless procedure carried out in a few minutes on an outpatient basis.

You lie on a couch with your neck stretched back. There is a slight prick as a fine needle is inserted into the thyroid gland and a small sliver of tissue removed. Some doctors first inject a local anaesthetic to anaesthetize the skin and underlying fatty tissue over the site to be biopsied but many patients find this unnecessary. Some doctors use a large bore needle or even a drill with previous local anaesthetic and, although it is a little frightening having something pushed into your neck, it does not really hurt. After the biopsy a small plaster dressing is put over the puncture mark in your neck and you can safely go home after a short rest.

Unfortunately not enough tissue may be obtained for the pathologist, who examines the cells, to make a firm diagnosis and sometimes the cells are not taken from the abnormal area. If there is continuing doubt your doctor may advise you to have an 'open' or surgical biopsy. This amounts to a formal surgical operation and provides both a firm diagnosis and often a cure because the whole of the lump in question and the surrounding tissue are removed.

X-rays

Conventional X-ray pictures may be used to assess whether an enlarged thyroid gland is pressing on your windpipe or, if the goitre is larger on one side than the other, whether the windpipe is being displaced. A retrosternal or a mediasternal thyroid may first be discovered only by chance from an X-ray of your chest taken for some other purpose. The nature of the retrosternal shadow may have to be confirmed by an isotope scan.

Computer-assisted tomography (a 'CAT' or 'CT' scan) of the eyes and the bony sockets in which they lie is helpful to establish the nature of the eye changes that may be associated with Graves' disease, especially when these changes are confined to only one eye (Plate 5).

Questions and Answers

Q. 1   Will I have a lot of blood tests that will hurt?

A.   It is unlikely that more than one or two samples of blood will be taken from a vein. Many tests can be done on one sample. The taking of a blood sample is not usually painful.

Q. 2   How will my doctor be able to tell if I have an overactive or an underactive thyroid?

A.   He may know from your symptoms and his findings, but he will confirm the diagnosis by tests. It is likely that he will measure the levels of your thyroid-stimulating hormone (TSH) and your thyroxine (T_4) to decide. He may also measure, on the same sample, your triiodothyronine (T_3) level if he thinks you are thyrotoxic.

*Q.*3   Is thyrotoxicosis the same thing as thyroid overactivity and hyper-thyroidism?

A.   Yes. All these terms mean your thyroid is producing excessive amounts of thyroid hormones.

*Q.*4   Does it mean I have cancer if I'm given a radioactive iodine test?

A.   Absolutely not.

*Q.*5   Are there several causes for overactivity or underactivity of the thyroid gland?

A.   Yes. In Chapters 5 and 6 the causes of hyperthyroidism are discussed and in Chapter 8 the causes of hypothyroidism.

*Q.*6   What are thyroid auto-antibodies?

A.   They are chemicals produced in your body that influence your thyroid cells. They may destroy them or they may stimulate them (pp. 11 and 22).

*Q.*7   If I have an isotope scan will it impair my fertility?

A.   No, it won't—not at all. The dose of irradiation is less than that given when a simple chest X-ray is done.

*Q.*8   Why is my hospital doctor so keen on finding out why I have an overactive thyroid gland?

A.   Because the most effective treatment depends upon the cause.

*Q.*9   What does the doctor at the hospital mean when he says that I'm to have a biopsy done as an outpatient?

A.   A needle biopsy is a procedure to remove a small piece of tissue from your thyroid gland; it is a simple procedure for which there is no need to stay in hospital.

*Q.*10 Shouldn't I have had some X-rays taken?

A.   X-rays are of limited value in the investigation of thyroid diseases, so don't worry if X-rays haven't been done.

4

Overactivity of the thyroid due to Graves' disease

Overactivity of the thyroid gland, also known as hyperthyroidism or thyrotoxicosis, is a disease in which increased amounts of usually both thyroid hormones, thyroxine (T_4) and triiodothyronine (T_3), are present in the bloodstream. In about 10 per cent of people with thyroid over-activity, only the T_3 level is raised, but the symptoms and the findings are just the same in this so-called T_3-toxicosis.

The causes of thyroid overactivity

The causes for overactivity of the thyroid are several (Table 2) but in practice more than 80 per cent of cases are due to the gland being made overactive by thyroid-stimulating antibodies. This condition is called Graves' disease or diffuse toxic goitre. It is 'diffuse' because the whole gland is overactive, as can be shown by an isotope scan (p. 23), and you are 'toxic' because you are ill—not sick because of some abnormal 'toxin' but because the cells of your body are being over-stimulated by the increased levels of thyroid hormones circulating in your bloodstream.

In this chapter only Graves' disease is considered. The other less common causes of thyroid overactivity are discussed in Chapter 6.

Table 2   Some of the common causes of hyperthyroidism

- Graves' disease (diffuse toxic goitre)
- Multinodular toxic goitre
- Toxic adenoma
- Viral thyroiditis
- Hashitoxicosis
- Excessive dosage with T_4 or T_3

Causes of Graves' disease

Several factors are involved in causing Graves' disease:

- Often there is a familial or hereditary factor because auto-immune diseases tend to run in families (Chapter 15).
- The dietary intake of iodine is relevant because the disease often presents in the spring and summer after an increase in iodine intake during the previous months.
- Females at all ages are some ten to fifteen times more likely than males to develop the condition. What triggers off the disease in those who are susceptible is unknown.
- In some instances Graves' disease seems to follow an emotional upset but it has not been possible to establish proof of such a cause-and-effect relationship. For example during the present troubles in Northern Ireland which started in 1968 there has been no significant increase in the incidence of Graves' disease. Nevertheless there is experimental evidence that an emotional upset may disturb the auto-immune system.
- The fundamental cause of Graves' disease is the formation of anti-bodies that stimulate the thyroid cells to excess activity.

Who gets Graves' disease?

The disease is most common in women aged 20–40, but it may occur in younger girls of 5 or more and very rarely in a baby born of a mother who has, or has had in the past, Graves' disease (p. 101). It may also occur in older patients of either sex and then presents in a rather different form from that in the younger patient.

What does it feel like?

The condition may come on insidiously, and it may be several months before you realize that you are ill. Tiredness is often an early symptom, to be followed by weight loss, palpitations or consciousness of your heart, nervousness and particularly irritability so that you have 'a short fuse', and increased sweating. Looseness of the bowels is not uncommon and sometimes diarrhoea may be a prominent symptom, causing diagnostic difficulties unless the other features are detected.

You will feel hot and be uncomfortable in hot weather. You may complain that the central heating is set too high or throw off the bed-clothes at night, yet your partner complains it is not *that* hot. Your skin may itch but there is no rash.

The tiredness gets worse and you may find yourself short of breath, particularly if you hurry while carrying shopping bags or climbing stairs. You may have a better than normal appetite; indeed you may be very hungry all the time. Even with this voracious appetite you are likely to lose weight—7-20 lb (3-9.5 kg) in a few months. Your periods will tend to become less heavy and you may miss a period or they may stop altogether. If this happens young women may wonder if they are pregnant but in fact they are likely to be infertile, a problem that corrects itself when the thyroid overactivity is brought under control.

You may not recognize that you are physically weak. The muscles in the upper part of your legs and arms are most likely to be affected. You may have difficulty in getting up from the squatting position without using your arms or find it hard to lift a heavy package down from a high shelf.

The older patient with Graves' disease.   In patients aged 55 or over the typical features described above may be less apparent and the brunt of the disease tends to fall upon the heart. The older patient often presents with shortness of breath, swollen ankles, and a fast irregular heart beat which is called atrial fibrillation. Sleeping may be difficult unless you are propped up in bed and you may find by chance that it is easier to sleep sitting up in an armchair. The cause of this heart failure may not always be immediately apparent.

Curiously some old people with Graves' disease become 'bloated' and lugubrious; they are slowed down and depressed (so-called 'apathetic hyperthyroidism', see p. 108).

Eye complications

The first thing you may notice is that something is wrong with your eyes. You may see in the mirror, or your friends may tell you, that one or both of your eyes has become starey. The upper lids are pulled upwards and the white of the eyes is more obvious (so-called 'lid retraction'). Because of this upper lid elevation your eyes appear larger (Plate 6). The appearance is rather like an actress trying to convey fear or horror. This appearance may occur in thyroid overactivity from any cause, not only Graves' disease. It improves as the overactivity of the thyroid gland is controlled or cured.

In Graves' disease, however, further eye troubles may arise, and these are discussed in Chapter 5.

Skin changes

You may notice that your skin is becoming thinner and more delicate, but this is seldom very obvious. Occasionally people with Graves' disease, and particularly those in whom the eye changes are marked, develop a curious change in the skin on their lower legs. Patches develop that are slightly reddened and thickened so that they stand up above the surrounding normal skin (Plate 7). Hair growing in the affected areas becomes coarser. The areas tend to increase in size and new ones may appear on the top of your foot or on the big toe. This condition is called *pretibial myxoedema*.

What does your doctor find when he examines you?

You are likely to be thin or at least show evidence of weight loss. You may be restless and anxious. You may not have noticed it but it is hard for you to sit still and you probably fidget, plucking at your handbag or twiddling your fingers (Fig. 4). Children tend to be clumsy and drop things; they may have grown faster than their contemporaries so that their height is greater than normal for their age.

Even on a cold day you will probably be lightly clad. The palms of your hands are hot and moist and your pulse bounding. Medical students are sometimes told, 'if you want to know the thyroid status of a young lady, you only have to hold her hand!' When your doctor asks you to hold out your arms in front of you and close your eyes, he may notice a fine tremor of your fingers. Your pulse rate is likely to be fast: this may be due in part to 'natural' nervousness on your part, but in fact the fast rate is persistent and present even when you are asleep. Sometimes, particularly in the older patient, the heart beat is irregular due to atrial fibrillation.

Your thyroid gland may be normal in size but usually it is slightly enlarged, sometimes sufficiently so for a goitre to be your presenting complaint. Because it is overactive, the blood flow through the gland is increased and this may be audible as a swishing noise when your doctor

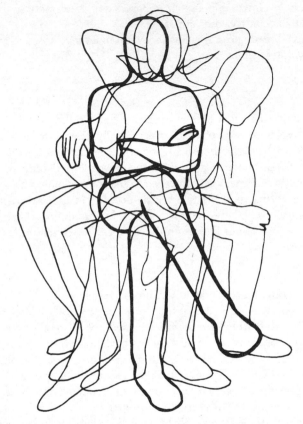

Fig. 4 A representation of a patient with thyroid overactivity (thyrotoxicosis). Notice the restlessness. The patient cannot sit still and fidgets.

puts a stethoscope on the front of your neck and asks you to stop breathing for a moment.

Often your eyes have a staring quality and this may be the first outward visible sign that alerts the doctor to what is wrong with you. Although you may be unaware that your muscles are weak, this can be obvious to your doctor. The most affected muscles are those round the shoulder and pelvic girdles. This weakness is more common in men than women. You may be surprised to find that you cannot raise your outstretched arms against the slight resistance of the doctor's hands or it may be difficult for you to get up from a squatting or lying position.

Confirming the diagnosis

In its earliest stages, overactivity of the thyroid may not be easy to diagnose. Later when the picture is more florid, it is easier. Your doctor has to distinguish thyroid overactivity from anxiety. Certainly in the younger person hyperthyroidism is virtually always accompanied by some feelings and evidence of anxiety, and the problem for the doctor is to distinguish anxiety alone from hyperthyroidism *plus* anxiety. The physical accompaniments of thyroid overactivity such as the weight loss, the fine tremor of the hands, and other evidence of increased metabolism are usually more pronounced than in uncomplicated anxiety, and laboratory tests will make the distinction.

The older patient who presents with heart failure must be recognized as suffering from thyroid overactivity, because with prompt treatment the outlook is good and often better than for certain other forms of heart failure.

Laboratory tests usually give clear-cut confirmation of the diagnosis. The total or free T_4 and the total or free T_3 levels are raised above normal and the TSH level is depressed. In the early stages only your T_3 level may be raised but the TSH level will be depressed.

When the laboratory results are only marginally abnormal, little is lost if your doctor keeps you under observation and uses time as a diagnostic ally. The clinical picture and the laboratory tests will become clearer a month or two later.

Once a diagnosis of hyperthyroidism has been made by your doctor, he or she will wish to determine whether you have Graves' disease or one of the several other causes of thyrotoxicosis shown in Table 2 and discussed in Chapter 6.

A diagnosis of Graves' disease may be obvious if you have the characteristic eye changes associated with the condition and is even more likely if there is a history of thyroid disease in your family. It may be clear to your doctor from your history and the tenderness of your thyroid that you have got subacute viral thyroiditis (Chapter 9). Difficulties arise, however, if you have silent thyroiditis (p. 107). Examination of your neck may suggest that causes other than Graves' disease are the reason for the thyroid overactivity because one or more nodules are found in the gland.

In Graves' disease an isotope scan will show an increased uptake of the radioisotope uniformly throughout both lobes. Furthermore, nearly all patients with Graves' disease have thyroid-stimulating antibodies (thyrotrophin-receptor antibodies) in their blood, but this test is not universally available.

How will you be treated?

Curative treatment

If you have got Graves' disease treatment is essential. In the old days about 20 per cent of untreated patients used to die and others ran a long fluctuating course with temporary remissions and relapses.

There are three main methods, not mutually exclusive, of treating Graves' disease. These are:

- antithyroid drugs which suppress the ability of the thyroid gland to make thyroid hormones but induce a permanent cure in only about 50 per cent of patients;
- radio-iodine, ^{131}I, which is concentrated in the thyroid cells and by irradiation destroys them;
- surgical removal of most of the thyroid gland (subtotal thyroidectomy).

Which of these methods is used depends on several factors and circumstances which must be discussed between you and your doctor. The more important of these are:

- whether your hyperthyroidism is due to Graves' disease, or some other condition. All three methods can be used if you have got Graves' disease;
- your age;
- your sex;
- whether the thyroid gland is large or not, whether it is cosmetically unsightly, and whether it is causing compression or displacement of the windpipe;
- whether the thyroid gland is in the normal position or is lying behind the sternum;
- whether it is convenient for you to remain under medical supervision for treatment with antithyroid drugs or whether you want a rapid, once-and-for-all cure;
- whether an experienced thyroid surgeon is available because his results are likely to be better than those of a surgeon who does only occasional thyroid surgery;

- what previous treatment, if any, you have had. For example, if you have relapsed after a previous course of medical treatment, a second course of antithyroid drugs is unlikely to achieve a permanent cure. If you have had surgery and thereafter relapsed, further surgery is contra-indicated because the incidence of postoperative complications is too high;
- financial considerations. Surgical treatment with a week-long stay in hospital and the surgeon's and anaesthetist's fees is more expensive than treatment with radio-iodine. A year or 18 months of medical treatment is less expensive than surgery but more expensive than radio-iodine.

It is important for your peace of mind that you understand these considerations and appreciate the risks and the advantages and disadvantages of each form of treatment which are discussed further in this chapter.

Non-curative treatment

Two forms of treatment that will improve your symptoms and make you feel better, but will not permanently cure the overactivity of the thyroid gland, are important.

Beta-adrenergic blocking drugs, colloquially known as beta-blockers, reduce your sweating, the anxiety and restlessness, your palpitations and your fast heart-rate, and the tremor of your hands. Propranolol is commonly used for this purpose and in general is a very safe drug. However it should not be taken by people who are prone to asthma. The tablets have to be taken two or three times daily. There are other beta-blockers with slightly different modes of action and some of these are taken only once daily. Your doctor may decide that one of these is more appropriate for you than propranolol. The beta-blockers make you feel more comfortable until a proper cure has been achieved, but do not by themselves cure the condition. It is important for you to know that treatment with a beta-blocker should never be stopped suddenly, and you must not let yourself run out of tablets. When there is no more need for a beta-blocker, the dosage will be gradually reduced over a week or 10 days before the drug is finally stopped.

Iodine has a temporary suppressive effect on the thyroid gland, but this lasts for only 3 or 4 weeks. In the present-day management of hyper-thyroidism iodine is reserved for making you ready for surgery. You may be asked to take it in the form of drops of iodine (Lugol's iodine) in a little milk three times daily or as tablets for 7–14 days before your operation.

Antithyroid drugs

A number of drugs suppress the synthesis of the thyroid hormones, reduce hormone production and will render you euthyroid. If the drug is given in too large a dose over too long a period of time you may become hypothyroid. Thus the dosage must be adjusted by your doctor, who may start with a large dose and later reduce it, and regulate it by your clinical response and the blood hormone level. Once the hyperthyroidism has been brought under control, it is simpler for you to take a moderate dose of the antithyroid drug continuously and prevent hypothyroidism developing by taking, in addition, a small dose of thyroxine. This may seem paradoxical but it prevents you from having the ups and downs of being over- and underactive as may happen if the dosage of the anti-thyroid drug is constantly being adjusted. Another reason for giving a moderate dose of the antithyroid drug, and using thyroxine to prevent thyroid underactivity developing, is that there is evidence that anti-thyroid drugs have a beneficial effect on the auto-immune process that is going on in your thyroid gland.

Although antithyroid drugs will certainly render you euthyroid, they may not provide a permanent cure. When the drug is stopped, the thyroid overactivity may gradually return over the next 3–24 months. In Graves' disease, treatment for 12–18 months is associated with a permanent remission in only about 50 per cent of patients. We are not sure why some people respond so favourably whereas others, in a matter of months or years after stopping treatment, have a return of their thyroid overactivity.

People who achieve a permanent remission often have mild thyro-toxicosis, with a normal sized or only slightly enlarged gland and are treated from an early stage. Conversely those who have a large and vascular gland, are severely thyrotoxic and treatment is started late are more liable to relapse when the antithyroid drug is stopped. But the size and vascularity of the gland and the severity of the hyperthyroidism are certainly not the only factors that determine the long-term response to antithyroid drugs. Your genetic constitution may be important and so also is the level of the thyroid-stimulating antibodies when the course of treatment has been completed.

You must not look upon a relapse after medical treatment as a disaster. It simply prolongs the period of medical supervision until you are rendered euthyroid by subtotal thyroidectomy or radio-iodine treatment. Which of these is used largely depends on your preferences but in most instances radio-iodine may then prove the treatment of choice.

People often ask why they cannot have another course of antithyroid drugs. They can, but experience has shown that failure to induce a permanent remission after the first course is almost invariably followed by a relapse after a second or even a third course. Nor is protracted treatment with antithyroid drugs a good idea because the intensity of the underlying disease fluctuates from time to time and this means you must be under prolonged medical supervision.

Antithyroid drugs are best not used for treating people whose job precludes them from regular medical supervision, nor for those who cannot be relied upon to take their tablets regularly. If you want a quicker once-and-for-all cure choose radio-iodine or surgery. Surgery is indicated when the goitre is large and unsightly because the gland may not shrink in size very much after radio-iodine. Surgery is probably best when the goitre is retrosternal or when it is causing displacement or compression of the windpipe, particularly if of sufficient degree to interfere with your breathing (p. 42).

There is some evidence that a rapid reduction in the thyroid hormone levels may aggravate the eye complications. For this reason initial treatment with antithyroid drugs is often used to assess the effect on your eyes before deciding whether to go ahead with definitive curative treatment in the form of radio-iodine or surgery.

Age. Antithyroid drugs are used for those rare cases of hyperthyroidism occurring in new-born babies (Chapter 13). It is also probably the best treatment for children with Graves' disease, although they seldom experience a permanent remission. If you have a daughter with an overactive thyroid, antithyroid drugs with additional thyroxine to keep her euthyroid will probably be used until she reaches the age of about 18 years. Then, when she has finished school and before she goes to university or starts work, definitive treatment with radio-iodine or surgery can be used.

Sex. Antithyroid drugs are commonly used for treating women aged

20–40 who have developed mild Graves' disease with a normal sized gland or a small goitre, and who have a 50 per cent chance of having a permanent remission. However, this may not be the optimal treatment if you are contemplating starting a family in the near future. Although hyperthyroidism often reduces the frequency of menstruation and induces temporary infertility, antithyroid treatment will quickly correct this situation. Therefore while having antithyroid treatment you may become pregnant. This does not present an insurmountable problem, because during pregnancy the antithyroid drug in low dosage can be given without danger to the baby inside you, provided that the treatment is stopped 4–6 weeks before the baby is born. Having had the baby, you will need to restart the antithyroid medication but as this may be secreted in your milk, breast-feeding is not usually advised, although the amounts are so small they are unlikely to harm the baby. Life is not made easier for you, if in addition to have to look after your new baby, you have to go to the doctor to have the treatment of your Graves' disease supervised. These difficulties can largely be avoided if radio-iodine or surgery is used in young women facing the prospect of having children, although it is customary to advise against pregnancy for 1 year after radio-iodine treatment and it is best avoided unless reliable contraception (the 'pill') is used.

What are the antithyroid drugs? The three most commonly used are carbimazole, methimazole, and propylthiouracil. Carbimazole and methimazole are closely related and the former is quickly converted to the latter in the body. Carbimazole is widely used in Europe and methimazole in North America. Propylthiouracil, which your doctor may call PTU, can be looked upon nowadays as a second-line drug that is used if side-effects occur with one of the other two.

Have they got side-effects? Yes, but they are not common. Nevertheless if you are prescribed an antithyroid drug it is important that you know about them. The side-effects usually occur, if they are going to occur at all, during the first 2 months of treatment. In order of frequency, carbimazole or methimazole may cause nausea or mild indigestion and skin rashes. Next, and less common, may come the unusual combination of pain in the joints, a low-grade fever, and sometimes swelling of the lymphatic glands. These reactions disappear quickly when the drug is stopped and may not recur if propylthiouracil is used as an alternative.
    The most serious side-effect of any of these three preparations is a

reduction in the white corpuscles in your blood. This reaction, which happens less frequently than 1 in 1000 cases, usually occurs, if at all, during the first few weeks of treatment. For unknown reasons—and fortunately it is very rare—the antithyroid drug may prevent the bone marrow making a particular type of white corpuscle, the granulocyte or neutrophil, and the number of these cells may fall (neutropenia) or they may disappear from the blood almost completely (agranulocytosis). These cells are essential for fighting off any micro-organisms that may invade your body. Usually the first manifestation of neutropenia or agranulocytosis is a sore throat. If you are taking an antithyroid drug and develop a nasty sore throat it is essential for you to stop taking the tablets immediately, and within 12 hours you should see your doctor or go to the hospital where you are being treated so that a white corpuscle count can be done. If this shows that the neutrophils (granulocytes) are depleted, penicillin is usually given to kill off the invading organisms until such time as your bone marrow has recovered and the white corpuscles have returned to your bloodstream in normal numbers. If you are sensitive to penicillin, some other appropriate antibiotic can be used.

Radio-iodine treatment

In many respects this is a very convenient method for treating Graves' disease. The advantages of radio-iodine are:

- you take it by mouth as a capsule or a number of capsules as an outpatient;
- you do not have to be admitted to hospital;
- you avoid, as compared with surgery, an anaesthetic, the pain of an operation and a scar on your neck;
- depending on the dose of radio-iodine given, you are likely to be off work for only one to three days unless your job involves contact with radio-sensitive materials or close proximity to other people;
- it is cheaper than surgery.

Radio-iodine has been used in the treatment of Graves' disease for 50 years and has proved itself safe. There have been no adverse effects from the irradiation such as the later development of leukaemia, no lack of fertility, and no genetic abnormalities in offspring. Nevertheless it is not given if you are pregnant because from the third month of pregnancy the thyroid gland of the fetus takes up iodine and hence your baby's thyroid would be irradiated too. Nor is radio-iodine usually used for the treatment of patients less than 18 years of age unless there is some special reason.

What then are the disadvantages? You may have slight soreness of the neck for a few days. Then there is the inconvenience that after you have been given your dose of radio-iodine you are radioactive for a short time. Most of this radioactivity will be eliminated in your urine within 48 hours and normal sanitary arrangements are perfectly adequate to cope with this. Depending on the dose you are given, you should not kiss anyone and you should not get closer than a metre to babies or children for 7 to 14 days. Nor for the first day or two after treatment with conventional doses should you be in close proximity with other adults for a long time, particularly those of child-bearing age. Your physician will advise you about this and will probably give you a card of instructions. Travel by private transport is perfectly safe after the conventional doses of radio-iodine used for treating thyrotoxicosis and travel by public transport has very few restrictions.

Another surmountable disadvantage is that, although radio-iodine has some early effect on the making of the thyroid hormones by the thyroid cells, its maximum effect is not apparent for about 3 months. In other words its action is slower than that of antithyroid drugs which produce a noticeable improvement in a week or two. While waiting for the radio-iodine to work you can be kept comfortable from the symptomatic point-of-view with a beta-blocker. In severe cases of thyrotoxicosis antithyroid drugs are given after the radio-iodine until it has produced its maximum beneficial effect.

The major disadvantage of radio-iodine, which must be weighed against its many advantages, is the liability for the thyroid to become underactive in the ensuing years. During a period of 2–20 years, more than 80 per cent of patients with Graves' disease become thyroid deficient after ^{131}I treatment and the incidence is not materially influenced by the dose of radio-iodine, although the larger the dose the earlier the underactivity comes on.

This disadvantage is less of a practical problem than you might think, although many women are understandably horrified at the prospect that they might become fat and bloated as a result of thyroid deficiency. This will not be allowed to happen. Provided you are kept under observation the chances of you experiencing thyroid deficiency are small, because replacement therapy with thyroxine can be started as soon as the TSH level starts to rise—before you notice any physical changes. Many clinics follow-up their patients who have been treated with radio-iodine by an annual postal questionnaire, with or without a blood test, but ideally you should see your doctor every year and have a blood test done.

Judging the correct dose of radio-iodine is difficult for the doctor. If too little is given, you will remain thyrotoxic and will need a second or more doses. If too much is given, the sooner will you become hypothyroid, but with close observation this will be countered by giving you thyroxine replacement treatment. In some centres the dose is calculated by the size of the thyroid gland and its avidity in taking up a tracer dose of isotope. In others the philosophy is to accept that, sooner or later, you are likely to become hypothyroid and therefore why not give a sizeable dose of ^{131}I and prescribe thyroxine as soon as the TSH level rises. This has the advantage that you will not worry about becoming hypothyroid and you will not have to be followed-up so often.

Therefore in accepting radio-iodine treatment for your Graves' disease, you should also accept the likelihood of needing thyroxine replacement therapy in due course, but this is not inevitable.

Surgery

In skilled hands surgical removal of most of the thyroid gland is a very effective form of treatment for Graves' disease. Before the operation you must first be rendered euthyroid either with iodine or an antithyroid drug—usually both. It is dangerous to operate on a thyrotoxic patient because this may provoke a thyroid crisis (p. 108). Although some surgeons operate when the patient's symptoms have only been improved with a beta-blocker, this is not a practice we subscribe to because you are not euthyroid.

In the hands of an experienced surgeon and a skilled anaesthetist you are unlikely to be in hospital longer than a week. Although the appearance of the scar can never be guaranteed, in most instances it eventually becomes a fine line that looks like a crease in your neck and the cut in the skin is made across the neck in one of the natural creases already there. Techniques from plastic surgery are used to close the wound after some seven-eighths of the gland have been removed. Most surgeons tend deliberately to remove rather too much than too little. This is to avoid leaving too much of the gland with the risk that the remnant is sufficiently large to sustain a recurrence of your hyperthyroidism. If this should happen, a second operation, although possible, is best avoided as second operations are followed by an increased incidence of complications (see below). If there is a post-operative recurrence, radio-iodine is used in patients of any age or sex to cure the thyrotoxicosis.

Surgical treatment is usually preferred if:

- the goitre is retrosternal;
- it is cosmetically unsightly; or
- it is compressing or displacing the windpipe.

If you have pressure on the trachea you may experience some difficulty in breathing, but before this happens you may make a curious crowing noise when you are asleep, and this may alarm your partner. This stridor, as it is called, occurs as your head slumps forwards or to one side when you are fast asleep, and the relaxed neck muscles allow the enlarged thyroid gland to compress the windpipe even more. Antithyroid drugs or radio-iodine are best avoided under these circumstances because either treatment may temporarily increase the size of the goitre and aggravate the degree of compression.

In 20 per cent or more of surgically-treated patients hypothyroidism develops post-operatively. The surgeon cannot be blamed for this because he has rightly veered towards removing too much rather than too little of the gland. After the operation you will be followed-up and if thyroid underactivity is going to develop as a direct consequence of the surgery this is usually apparent within 3 months. Thyroid deficiency may also develop later on because of auto-immune destruction of your thyroid cells. If this happens it is easily treated by taking thyroxine tablets by mouth to make good the deficit.

Other complications of surgery

Two other complications may follow surgery but both are extremely rare.

Trouble with your voice. Running in or near the thyroid gland on either side of the neck are the nerves that activate the vocal cords (the recurrent laryngeal nerves). If these are bruised at the time of the operation you may have a hoarse voice afterwards, although some huskiness is not uncommon for a day or two simply as a result of the anaesthetic. Permanent hoarseness will occur only if one of the nerves to the vocal cords is actually cut, but this seldom happens with an experienced thyroid surgeon using modern techniques.

Muscle cramps. The other possible post-operative complication is related to damage to the parathyroid glands. Usually there are four of these pea-sized glands (two on each side) which lie towards the back of the thyroid gland and they may be hidden in it. The surgeon makes every endeavour not to damage these and it is most unusual for the blood supply to all four to be permanently cut off. But they may be bruised during the operation and therefore may not function normally for some days or weeks afterwards.

The parathyroid glands regulate the level of calcium in your blood. If they do not function properly the level of calcium falls and this may give rise to a condition called tetany. In the unlikely event of this happening to you, the first thing you may notice is a feeling of numbness of your lips and round your mouth. Later you may experience cramp in the hands and sometimes in the feet. These symptoms are corrected by giving you calcium and vitamin D, or one of its related compounds, to restore your blood calcium level to normal. Usually this treatment is necessary for only a short time.

Treatment of pretibial myxoedema

The course of pretibial myxoedema is unpredictable. Almost invariably it occurs in patients who have rather bad eye problems. As your hyper-thyroidism responds to treatment so the skin changes in the legs may improve. In some patients, however, pretibial myxoedema does not occur until after your thyrotoxicosis has been cured.

The most effective treatment is to apply a potent corticosteroid oint-ment each night to the affected areas on your leg, rub it well in, and then wrap pieces of polythene film (Clingfilm, Saranwrap, Klingfilm) round the involved parts of the leg. This treatment may have to continue for quite a long time (Plate 7).

A few words of comfort

Graves' disease is not an easy disease for anyone to bear with. You will appreciate that whether you are treated with antithyroid drugs, radio-iodine or surgery there is no *immediate* instant cure. It is upsetting to have to take antithyroid drugs for a period as long as 12 to 18 months. Radio-iodine does not produce its maximum effect for 3 months. If you elect to have surgery, it will be necessary for you to be prepared for this because you must be rendered euthyroid before the operation is done. Even when you are better, follow-up is necessary, sometimes for the rest of your life.

The emotional or psychological accompaniments of Graves' disease are very real. Do not blame yourself if you are unduly anxious or find yourself irritable. This problem will pass, but you must be patient.

Matters are made worse if you suffer from the eye complications of Graves' disease (Chapter 5). These can be more worrying to a woman than any other aspect of the condition. Here too you must try to be patient. Plastic surgery may greatly improve the appearance of your eyes but this is usually not done until the thyroid overactivity has been cured.

Questions and Answers

*Q.*1   It doesn't mean I have cancer if my Graves' disease is treated with radio-iodine, does it?

A.   Graves' disease is not a malignant or cancerous condition. The answer is absolutely no.

*Q.*2   I have four children. Will they also get thyroid overactivity?

A.   Not necessarily but there is a chance that they could develop some auto-immune thyroid disease—either Graves' disease or Hashimoto's thyroid-itis (see Chapters 7 and 15).

*Q.*3   Will I get fat after I'm treated?

A.   If you have lost weight, you will probably regain it. If you were not fat originally, there is no reason for you to become fat after you've been treated for thyroid overactivity.

*Q.*4   Will radio-iodine have any effect on any children I have later on?

A.   No.

*Q.*5   I can feel my heart pounding away at night, and sometimes this keeps me awake. Can anything be done to help this?

A.   Certainly. Treatment with a beta-blocker will probably stop this happening until your overactive thyroid gland has been brought under control.

*Q.*6   I used to love hot weather but now I can't stand it. We have booked a family holiday in Spain this August. Should we cancel it?

A.   It is now April and by August your thyroid will no longer be secreting an excessive amount of thyroid hormones. By then you will not mind the lovely weather in Spain. No, don't cancel your holiday.

*Q.*7   I'm very short-tempered with the kids and snap at my husband all the time. Can you give me anything to stop this? Usually I'm a pretty tolerant, even-tempered sort of person.

A.   Yes, we can give you a beta-blocker for a while but as your thyroid condition improves you will stop being so irritable and nervous.

*Q.*8   Which treatment is right for me?

A.   This depends upon your particular circumstances and the advantages and disadvantages of the three treatments we've already discussed. Let us weigh up the pros and cons so that you can decide on balance which treatment will suit you best.

*Q.*9   Won't surgery leave a nasty scar?

A.   Almost certainly not. Usually it gradually fades to become like another crease in your neck.

5

The eye changes associated with Graves' disease

The eye changes in thyroid overactivity generally

Eye changes are common in thyroid overactivity whatever its cause and fortunately in many people these are not too troublesome, although they will cause you concern. There is likely to be a tendency for your upper eyelids to be pulled upwards, exposing more of the whites of your eyes. Thus your relatives or friends may comment that your eyes have developed a staring quality, like an actress does when she wishes to convey an impression of fear. This is called lid-retraction (Plate 6). When you look down, the upper lids may be slow to follow the downward movement of your eyeballs—a condition called lid-lag (Plate 8). These changes tend to get better as the overactive thyroid is brought under control.

The eye changes peculiar to Graves' disease

More troublesome are the eye changes that may occur only in Graves' disease and also, but very seldom, in Hashimoto's thyroiditis. The relationship in time between the thyroid disease and the involvement of the eyes varies. Usually the eye changes occur simultaneously with the onset of your thyroid overactivity but sometimes they precede it. Less often the eyes may go wrong months or even years after your thyroid overactivity has been treated and cured.

When associated with thyroid disease—past, present, or future—the condition is known as dysthyroid or Graves' ophthalmopathy. However, sometimes the eye changes occur without there ever being any over-activity of the thyroid gland at all, and this condition is called ophthalmic Graves' disease.

The changes usually affect both eyes but sometimes only one eye is involved, or one eye more than the other.

What causes the eye changes in Graves' disease?

There is inflammation at the back of your eyeballs which lie in rigid bony sockets in your skull. The cause of this inflammation is probably an auto-immune reaction mainly directed at the muscles that move your eyes from side-to-side and up and down (the oculomotor muscles). Obviously the antibodies involved are not the same as those that upset the thyroid gland because the eye changes may occur independently of any change in thyroid function.

What may happen to your eyes?

The inflammation causes swelling of the tissues behind the eyeballs and increases the pressure in the rigid bony orbit. This leads to a number of problems which may occur separately or together, and do not progress in any predictable manner.

1. Your eyes may be pushed forwards, which is known as proptosis or exophthalmos. This makes them more prominent and staring (Plate 9). Your doctor may measure painlessly how far your eyes are pushed forward with an instrument called an exophthalmometer (Fig. 5).

2. The increased pressure in the orbits may impair the normal drainage of fluid from your eyes so that your upper eyelids become puffy and even more swollen if there is involvement of the glands above the eyes that form tears (Plate 9). Impaired drainage from your lower lids may lead to 'bags' forming under your eyes.

3. Because your eyes are pushed forward they are less protected by the eyelids and therefore more exposed to irritation from dust, wind, and infection. You may have a feeling of grittiness or pain in your eyes, which water a lot, so that almost unconsciously you keep dabbing your eyes with your hankie. The outer membranes covering your eyes may become inflamed and increase the pain. Often the eyes appear as if they were water-logged and they may become bloodshot at the outer corners (Plate 10).

4. The muscles that move your eyeballs in different directions may be affected so that the eyes cease to move as well as they normally do (ophthalmoplegia). Upward gaze is usually affected first and you may discover that you cannot look up without tilting your head back,

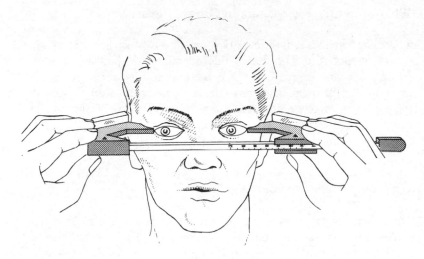

Fig. 5   An exophthalmometer being used to measure the degree of protrusion of the eyes.

which may cause an aching discomfort in the back of your neck. Later, movement of your eyes from side-to-side may be impaired. Because the eyeballs no longer move exactly in parallel with each other you develop double vision (diplopia). When looking straight ahead you will see a pencil held up straight in front of you by your doctor as one; however, when he moves the pencil upwards or to one side you see two pencils.

5. The increased pressure in your bony orbits may affect the optic nerves that carry the visual image from your eyes to the brain. This may threaten your eyesight.

Severe ophthalmopathy which may affect your vision is sometimes called 'malignant exophthalmos' (Plate 10). This is not a good term because the condition has nothing to do with cancer. Nevertheless it is serious and unless treated could lead to blindness.

How does the doctor know what is wrong?

The cause of the eye changes is usually obvious when your doctor finds you are thyrotoxic, but the diagnosis may be more difficult if you do not have thyroid overactivity, and particularly if the changes involve only one eye because other disorders in the orbit may produce the same appearances. The presence of thyroid auto-antibodies in your blood favours ophthalmic Graves' disease and about 60 per cent of people with this condition have thyroid-stimulating antibodies. Furthermore, the TSH level is often below the lower reference range despite the level of the thyroid hormones not being raised in ophthalmic Graves' disease.

Special X-rays or ultra-sound examination of the orbits may be needed to confirm the diagnosis. Computerized tomography (a CT- or CAT-scan) shows what is going on in the orbits by taking multiple sliced pictures of your eye sockets. In ophthalmopathy there is a characteristic thickening of the oculomotor muscles (Plate 5).

It is likely that you will have to see a specialist eye doctor who may carry out any one of a number of tests to:

- assess whether your general eyesight is all right;
- be sure that your ability to see different colours is normal;
- be sure that the membranes covering your eyeball are not damaged;
- measure the pressure in your eyeballs;
- see whether your fields of vision are normal; and
- chart the movements of your eyes to see that the eyeballs are moving properly in all directions and in parallel.

Treatment

If your eye problems are mild and do not get worse, you will probably not need any special treatment. For unknown reasons the eye changes are often worse in men (Plate 12) and also in those who smoke cigarettes.

In two-thirds of patients the stariness of the eyes caused by lid retraction diminishes as their thyroid overactivity is brought under control. The elevation of the upper lids may also be reduced by treatment with a beta-blocker. If the lid-retraction and lid-lag persist, plastic surgery to lower the position of the eyelids has a strikingly beneficial effect.

There is some evidence that treatment of the thyroid overactivity in Graves' disease with radio-iodine or surgery may aggravate the eye changes more than treatment with an antithyroid drug does. Although this has not been conclusively proven, many doctors believe it is prudent

to treat the Graves' disease medically to start with and see what effect
this has on your eyes. It is important to avoid making you thyroid
deficient because this may aggravate your eye problems.

When the eyes are swollen and feel gritty, methyl cellulose eye-drops
by day and a lubricating ointment at night often help. You may find that
your eyes are less puffy if you sleep propped up with several pillows.
Sometimes the temporary use of a diuretic tablet that increases the
elimination of fluid from the body helps. Your eyes may be more comfortable if you wear dark glasses with side pieces to protect them from the
wind and dust.

Double vision tends to improve in two-thirds of patients when their
thyroid overactivity is brought under control. Persistent double vision,
however, is a great nuisance and handicap. During the early phases you
may find that reading or watching television is made more tolerable
by wearing a patch over one eye. If you wear spectacles, painting clear
nail varnish over the inside of one lens will mean that you see only one
image. Alternatively special prisms can be supplied or fitted to your
existing spectacles to correct the double vision and allow you to drive
safely. Later when the condition of the eyes has become static, an eye
surgeon may correct the muscle imbalance so that the double vision is
permanently cured or at least improved.

A reduction in the protrusion of the eyes occurs spontaneously, but
slowly, in about 20 per cent of patients as the thyroid overactivity is
controlled. In more than half the patients it remains static and in about
20 per cent it becomes worse unless special treatment is given.

To reduce the protrusion of your eyes corticosteroids, akin to cortisone, can be effective as shown in Plates 13 and 14, and may be used in
conjunction with other drugs that suppress the auto-immune reaction
going on in your orbits. Sometimes you may be advised to have the outer
part of your eyelids sewn together under a local anaesthetic, because
by narrowing the opening between the eyelids, better coverage and
protection of your eyeballs is obtained and the cosmetic appearance is
improved.

Rarely, in less than 10 per cent of patients, is it necessary to enlarge
the bony orbits to allow the swollen tissue behind the eyeballs to expand
and thus reduce the pressure. Various surgical operations to achieve this
have been devised. Nowadays the floor of the bony orbit is usually
removed from inside the mouth without making any visible external
scar. The improvement from ocular discomfort, threatened vision, and in
cosmetic appearance can be striking (Plates 10 and 11).

The eye changes that may occur in Graves' disease are without doubt the most upsetting for any patient. The ophthalmopathy is difficult to treat and, sadly, despite the best treatments available at present, a proportion of patients may have persistent eye problems.

Questions and Answers

Q. 1   Do all patients with Graves' disease get eye problems?

A.   No, or only minor or temporary ones. Many thyrotoxic patients have no complaints about their eyes throughout the whole course of their illness.

Q. 2   Why am I not receiving any special treatment for my eyes?

A.   Your thyroid is still overactive, and hopefully your eyes will improve as your thyroid comes under control.

Q. 3   My eyes feel much less gritty this month and are watering less. Is this a good sign?

A.   Yes, this is what we like to see happen. There is likely to be further improvement.

Q. 4   I used to have nice eyes. Now they look terrible! I've got this puffiness over my upper eyelids and bags under my lower ones. What can I do about this?

A.   If you can, sleep propped up with more pillows. A diuretic to increase your urine output may also help. Try not to worry too much. Once your thyroid problem has been put right, we can consider other treatments for your eyes if they are still a problem.

Q. 5   Will my double vision ever clear up?

A.   Your eye condition may fluctuate independently of your thyroid hormone levels, although we hope your eyes will improve once everything else has settled down. If not then surgery to the eyes can be considered at a later date to ensure that at least you do not see double when looking straight ahead.

6

Other causes of thyroid overactivity

Although Graves' disease is the commonest cause of thyroid overactivity, you may become hyperthyroid under a number of other circumstances. These circumstances are listed below, roughly in the order of their frequency, although this varies in different parts of the world.

- A toxic multinodular goitre (see below);
- a solitary toxic 'hot' adenoma (p. 53);
- as a result of having subacute virus thyroiditis (see Chapter 9);
- in association with Hashimoto's thyroiditis, so called Hashitoxicosis (see Chapter 7);
- as a result of taking too much thyroxine, triiodothyronine, or thyroid extract by mouth (p. 53);
- thyroid overactivity induced by taking iodine-containing substances (p. 55);
- a thyroid cancer (see Chapter 12);
- a disorder of the pituitary gland that results in excess production of thyroid-stimulating hormone and hence thyroid overactivity (p. 105); and
- a tumour of the reproductive system (male or female) which secretes a hormone that stimulates the thyroid gland (p. 56).

In any of these situations your symptoms are likely to be much the same as in Graves' disease (p. 29 *et seq.*) except that the eye changes (ophthalmopathy) peculiar to auto-immune thyroid disease rarely, if ever, occur.

Toxic multinodular goitre

This condition, also known as Plummer's disease after the American physician who described it in 1913, tends to arise in the older patient who, for many years has had a goitre which has become lumpy or nodular. The symptoms resemble those of Graves' disease. An isotope scan shows that the nodules are overactive ('hot') and separated by areas of inactivity. Radio-iodine is usually the preferred treatment but if the gland is large and unsightly, it is probably best for you to have it removed surgically after due pre-operative preparation (p. 41).

A solitary toxic 'hot' adenoma

In this condition a clump of cells, a nodule or benign tumour (an adenoma), becomes overactive and in effect takes over the function of the whole gland. The result is that all the activity is located in one area, and the rest of the gland goes into a resting state because, through the feed-back mechanism, the secretion of TSH from the pituitary is switched off by the hormone output from the 'hot' nodule. The offending solitary adenoma can usually, but not always, be felt by your doctor. The rest of the thyroid gland may not be enlarged or may be smaller than normal. The condition is more common in middle-aged and older women. In its early stages the adenoma may not produce excess thyroid hormones but later the levels of T_4 and particularly T_3 are likely to rise and the TSH is suppressed. The key to the diagnosis is a radio-isotope scan which shows uptake in the solitary nodule (Plate 2), which is therefore 'hot', and there is little or no uptake by the rest of the gland.

Antithyroid drugs are effective but do not induce a permanent remission. You can have the 'hot' nodule removed surgically but probably the best treatment is a fairly large dose of radio-iodine. This destroys the 'hot' adenoma, and the remaining normal, but previously suppressed gland gradually resumes its normal function.

Taking too much thyroxine or triiodothyronine

People for a number of reasons may take too much thyroxine, triiodo-thyronine, or sometimes thyroid extract although the last is seldom used nowadays as it is an impure substance of variable potency. The thyroid hormone levels in your blood depend upon which of these drugs you are taking in excess. If you are taking too much thyroxine, the T_4 and probably the T_3 levels will be raised. If you are taking too much triiodo-thyronine, the T_3 level will be raised and the T_4 is low. If you are taking thyroid extract the thyroid hormone levels may be normal but the level of another substance, thyroglobulin, will be increased. Irrespective of which compound you are taking to excess, the TSH level, measured by a sensitive method, will be low or undetectable.

Treatment of thyroid deficiency

If your thyroid is underactive, too much thyroxine (or sometimes tri-iodothyronine) may be prescribed while your doctor is adjusting the replacement dosage. How the correct dosage is arrived at is discussed on p. 70.

Self-treatment

Some people like being hyperthyroid; it gives them a 'high' and they treat themselves with thyroid hormones. Sometimes they deny that they are doing so ('thyrotoxicosis factitia').

Obesity

Thyroid hormones are sometimes given to help people lose weight but this is not necessarily beneficial. If the dose is small, all that happens is that by the feed-back mechanism the output of TSH is reduced. The thyroid gland then puts out less hormone but the level of thyroid hormones in the bloodstream remains normal because of the hormone being taken by mouth. If the dosage is larger, then the thyroid hormone levels will rise; you will become hyperthyroid and this will have an adverse effect on your heart and on your bones (osteoporosis).

In the past people were sometimes told that they were obese because they were suffering from thyroid deficiency and they have taken thyroid hormones ever since. Usually the initial diagnosis was based on the results of the only tests available in those days and these were unreliable. The most sensitive test for confirming thyroid underactivity is to measure the TSH (p. 16)—a test that only became available some 15 to 20 years ago. Belief that the initial diagnosis was correct may have been heightened by you losing a few pounds of weight after starting the treatment. This happened because thyroid hormones promote the loss of fluid from the body, and it was the loss of water rather than of fat that was responsible for this early weight reduction. Any further weight loss was probably more due to you eating less rather than the thyroid hormone you were taking. It is important to emphasize that hypo-thyroidism is very rarely the sole cause of obesity.

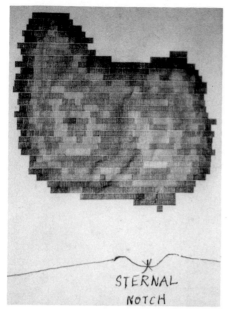

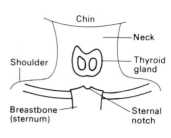

Plate 1. Normal technetium isotope scan of the thyroid gland. The outline of the gland is clearly shown. The right lobe is slightly larger than the left. The degree of uptake of the isotope is greatest in the centre of each lobe where there is the most thyroid tissue. The 'sternal notch' is the small hollow at the upper end of the breast-bone.

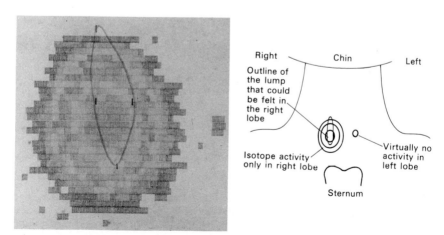

Plate 2. Technetium isotope scan of a thyroid gland containing a toxic adenoma. The 'hot' nodule in the right lobe takes up all the isotope, and there is virtually no radioactivity in the other lobe because it is inactive as a result of T_4 from the nodule suppressing the secretion of TSH from the pituitary gland (see text).

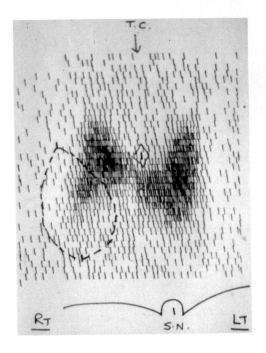

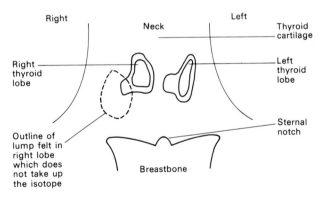

Plate 3. Technetium scan of the thyroid gland containing a 'cold' nodule. The outline of the nodule in the lower part of the right lobe, which could easily be seen and felt, has been inked in on the scan. There is no radioactivity in this nodule which is therefore 'cold'.

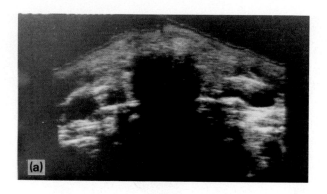

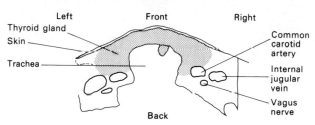

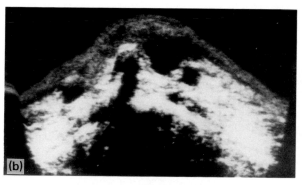

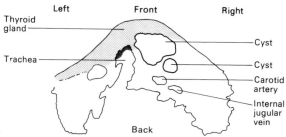

Plate 4. Ultrasound scans of the thyroid gland. (a) Normal. (b) A large and a small cyst in the right lobe are causing some thyroid enlargement.

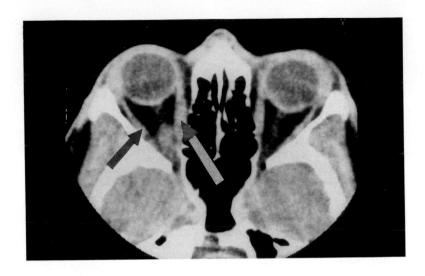

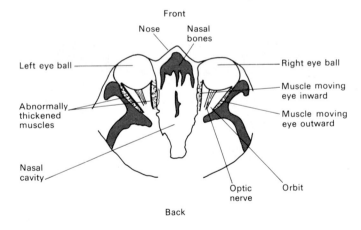

Plate 5. Computerized tomographic (CT) scan of the orbits, taken from above, in a patient with impaired movements of the left eye, and double vision when looking upwards and to the left. The eyeballs can be clearly seen, and some of the muscles (marked with an arrow) that move the left eyeball are thicker than those in the right orbit.

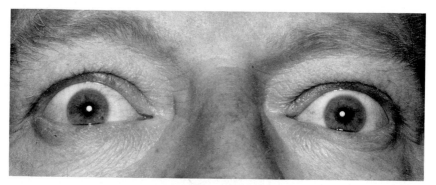

Plate 6. Lid retraction. Note how the upper eyelids are retracted so that the eyes have a staring quality and more of the white of the eyes than normal is visible.

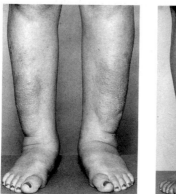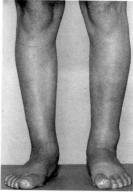

Plate 7. Pretibial myxoedema: (left) before treatment and (right) the appearance of the legs 18 months after the local application of corticosteroid ointment.

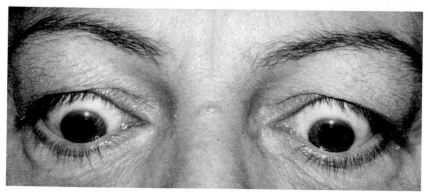

Plate 8. Lid lag. As the patient looks downwards, the upper lid lags behind the eyeball.

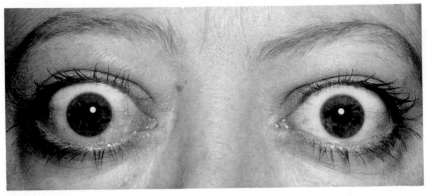

Plate 9. Exophthalmos or proptosis. Both eyeballs are more prominent than normal and protrude forwards. There is some swelling of the soft tissues above the upper eyelids. Note also that the eyes are somewhat bloodshot, the right more than the left.

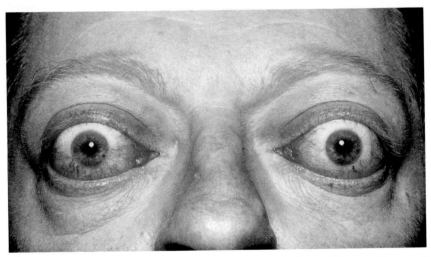

Plate 10. Marked ophthalmopathy showing exophthalmos, lid retraction, and increased redness.

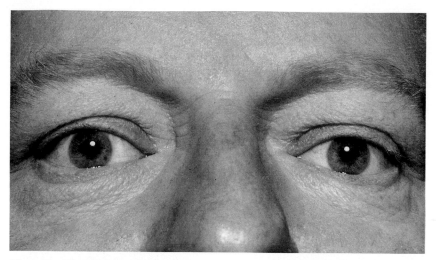

Plate 11. The same patient as in Plate 10 after two years' treatment including decompression of both orbits.

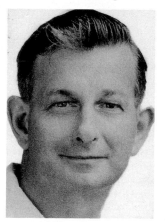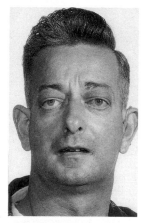

Plate 12. Appearance before (left) and after (right) the development of thyrotoxicosis.

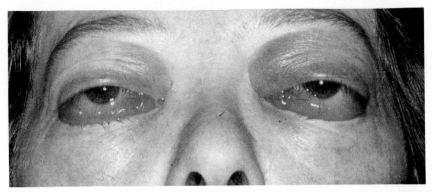

Plate 13. Severe ophthalmopathy in Graves' disease before treatment. The eyeballs are protruding forwards but the extent of this exophthalmos is in part masked by the swelling in and around the eyelids.

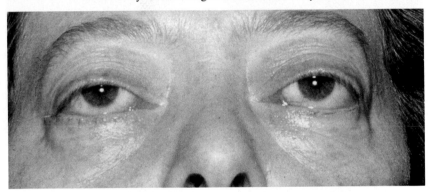

Plate 14. Ten days after treatment with prednisone (a corticosteroid drug) the ophthalmopathy (shown in Plate 13) is much improved. The eyes are less 'angry' and uncomfortable. The swelling of the eyelids is much reduced but upward movement of the eyeballs is still defective, which explains why the patient holds her head tilted back.

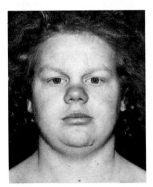 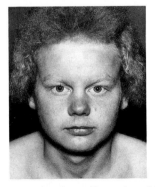

Plate 15. A 17-year-old carpenter with myxoedema (hypothyroidism): (left) before treatment; (right) after 18 months' treatment with thyroxine.

If you have been taking thyroxine for many years, it is important to know whether you really need this treatment, and if you do it may be necessary to adjust the dosage because as you grow older your thyroid deficiency may well become greater. Hence it is in your best interests if your doctor advises you to stop taking the hormone for 6–8 weeks and then have a modern sensitive test done to decide whether you really need it.

Iodine-containing substances

Certain medicines, substances ('dyes') used in special X-ray procedures (e.g. to show your kidneys or gall-bladder); and some 'health' foods such as Kelp may induce thyroid overactivity in susceptible people. These people usually live in an iodine-deficient part of the world and often have a pre-existing goitre. Radioisotope scanning may show that you have an increased uptake throughout the whole gland and therefore you have Graves' disease, or that you have one or more toxic adenomas.

In some instances the thyroid overactivity remits if the increased intake of iodine is stopped, and until this happens your symptoms can usually be controlled with a beta-blocker. In other people the hyperthyroidism persists and the condition is treated in the same way as Graves' disease or a toxic multinodular goitre.

Tumours that cause thyroid overactivity

These conditions are rare, but thyroid overactivity may occur in association with a number of different types of tumour.

Cancer of the thyroid gland which usually has spread to other parts of the body may cause hyperthyroidism. The presence of these overactive cells can be shown by a whole-body radio-iodine scan.

A tumour of your pituitary gland that secretes excess TSH will stimulate your thyroid to increased activity. Radio-iodine uptake by your thyroid gland will be increased but the TSH level will be normal or high, instead of being depressed or undetectable as it is in the much more common causes of thyroid overactivity.

A tumour of the ovary in which there is thyroid-like tissue may secrete excess T_4 and/or T_3. An isotope scan of the thyroid gland will show little or no uptake whereas one of the offending ovary will show a high uptake.

A tumour of the testis or ovary may produce a hormone that stimulates your thyroid gland. An isotope scan will show increased uptake by your thyroid, but usually the underlying tumour in the testis or ovary will already have produced local symptoms of which your doctor must be made aware.

The treatment of all these tumourous conditions is directed at the primary underlying cause.

Questions and Answers

Q.1   What exactly is a solitary toxic nodule?

A.   It is a cluster of thyroid cells that have taken over the function of the rest of your thyroid gland. This cluster of cells is now producing excessive amounts of thyroid hormones which is the reason why you feel so tired and have lost weight.

Q.2   Does a toxic nodule mean I have cancer?

A.   Certainly not.

Q.3   I have been taking 300 micrograms of thyroxine for 20 years—ever since my thyroid operation. Why have I been advised to reduce the dose?

A.   Three hundred micrograms is a large dose, and probably more than you need. Your recent thyroid hormone levels are very high and your TSH is undetectable, which confirms that you are having more thyroxine than you need. This is not good for your heart or for your bones. Your bones are probably getting weak from osteoporosis if you are going through the menopause and too much thyroxine will make the osteoporosis worse. Two hundred micrograms daily is usually sufficient to maintain normal thyroid hormone levels.

Q.4   I thought that iodine was good for you—so why has it been suggested that I should not take Kelp?

A.   Some iodine is needed by everyone, but not too much. In your case the thyroid has become overactive and the Kelp may be contributing.

*Q.*5 Will it stop being overactive when I stop taking Kelp?

A. It is impossible to be certain about this. If your thyrotoxicosis persists, then it can be treated.

*Q.*6 I have been told that I have an enlarged thyroid gland which is overactive and contains many nodules. I feel well but the swelling is unsightly and I think it is getting bigger. What can be done about the swelling?

A. If the gland is getting bigger and bothering you, particularly if it is beginning to press on surrounding structures, then surgical removal would be advisable.

7

Hashimoto's disease

Hashimoto's disease, Hashimoto's thyroiditis, or chronic lymphadenoid or lymphocytic goitre as it is sometimes called, is for several reasons an important condition.

1. It is common and affects about 1 woman in 10.
2. It is a significant cause of goitre especially in women—the female to male ratio being in excess of 10 to 1—and may affect female children and adolescents but is commoner in adults.
3. It is an important cause of thyroid underactivity (hypothyroidism). In many parts of the world it is the most common cause of thyroid deficiency although worldwide lack of iodine ranks first.

Cause of Hashimoto's disease

As explained in Chapter 2, Hashimoto's thyroiditis is an auto-immune disorder and seems to be caused by the presence of certain antibodies that react with the cells of the thyroid gland. Why these antibodies arise is not understood, but they develop more commonly in people with a particular genetic make-up and there is often a history of other auto-immune diseases in the patient's family or relatives (see Chapter 15). The so-called microsomal auto-antibodies, that appear in the blood and are formed by certain white corpuscles (lymphocytes), invade the thyroid gland and have the ability to destroy the thyroid cells but this is a very slow process.

Course of Hashimoto's disease

The course of the disease is often protracted over many years and during this time waxes and wanes in its destructive effect on the thyroid gland. At any stage the progression of the disease may appear to be arrested and to lie dormant. If you develop Hashimoto's thyroiditis, you may become aware of it and seek medical advice at many different stages along the road. For example the development of a small goitre may be in you the first manifestation of the disease. Alternatively and perhaps more commonly, you may not be aware that anything is wrong until late in the course of the condition when you become thyroid deficient.

A small proportion of people with Hashimoto's disease experience, usually early in the course of the disease, mild symptoms of thyroid overactivity (so-called Hashitoxicosis) for a few weeks or months. If you experience this, you will have the symptoms of Graves' disease and you may even have some of the eye changes of that condition (Chapters 4 and 5). Hashitoxicosis is due to thyroid-stimulating antibodies enhancing thyroid activity but the hyperthyroidism seldom lasts long because the thyroid destructive antibodies are the more powerful.

What do you feel?

In the early stages of Hashimoto's disease you will feel perfectly well but you or your family may notice that you have a small goitre. Later you may experience some discomfort in the front of your neck but there is no severe pain and the gland is simply tender on pressure. For a period of a month or two, often intermittently, you may have slight discomfort or a consciousness in your neck when you swallow.

If you are one of the few who have a temporary period of Hashitoxicosis, you will feel ill, lose weight, have pounding of the heart, feel overheated and be intolerant of hot weather. You may have looseness of your bowels, and your eyes may become starey. Indeed you may have any or all of the symptoms and signs of Graves' disease (Chapters 4 and 5).

Later in the course of the disease, as your thyroid gland functions less and less adequately, you will develop the symptoms of thyroid deficiency (Chapter 8) but these are often wrongly attributed to the menopause or you getting older.

How is the diagnosis confirmed?

Essentially the diagnosis of Hashimoto's disease is based on finding thyroid antibodies in your blood. The level of these often increases as the disease progresses. In the late stages when all the thyroid gland has been destroyed the level of the auto-antibodies may fall to low or undetectable levels.

The function of the thyroid gland has to be monitored at intervals throughout the long course of Hashimoto's disease because you may experience few if any symptoms until the hormone output of the gland begins to fail. Although treatment with thyroxine may prevent your goitre from becoming larger or may reduce its size, this therapy becomes essential when the T_4 level begins to fall. There has been debate as to whether treatment with thyroxine should be started before obvious overt hypothyroidism has appeared and when only the TSH level is raised and the T_4 level is normal (Chapter 8, Table 3). Some doctors find it logical to start treatment with thyroxine when there is evidence of impending thyroid failure as shown by a normal T_4 level but an unquestionably raised TSH and thyroid auto-antibodies. About 5 per cent per annum of such women become overtly hypothyroid and develop a low T_4. No harm comes from starting treatment early and you may find that you feel considerably better because with hind-sight you realize that you have been suffering from mild ill-health that crept up on you so silently that you did not notice it.

Treatment

We have no safe reliable way of modifying the faulty immunological system that mistakenly believes your thyroid cells are 'foreign'. Thus the basic cause of Hashimoto's thyroiditis is not treated.

If you have a temporary phase of Hashitoxicosis, a beta-blocker and/or antithyroid medication, such as carbimazole, may be given for a short time (p. 36). If the gland becomes uncomfortably painful a short course of corticosteroids may be used as in subacute viral thyroiditis (p. 76).

In general the treatment is the management of the consequences of thyroid failure, although a goitre is sometimes prevented from becoming larger or is reduced in size by giving thyroxine. The essential step is the prevention of hypothyroidism when this is imminent or the correction of hypothyroidism when this has developed. The best treatment is replacement therapy with thyroxine (p. 70).

Occasionally surgery is required, particularly if there is any possibility that the goitre is due to cancer and not to Hashimoto's disease. This difficulty may arise when the thyroid feels very hard or is enlarged unevenly, but usually a needle biopsy will resolve this diagnostic difficulty. Surgery is also advisable if you develop hoarseness of the voice, symptoms due to compression of the windpipe or the goitre is cosmetically unsightly despite treatment with thyroxine.

Nor should it be forgotten that Hashimoto's disease may be associated with other auto-immune diseases (Chapter 15), and it may be that you could develop one of these which will need treatment.

Let us follow Angela along the road of Hashimoto's disease, not forgetting that she started the condition long before we knew as much about it as we do now.

I'm now aged 60 and feel perfectly well. I take three thyroxine tablets every day—each tablet of 0.05 mg strength. When I was aged about 17, my mother noticed my thyroid gland was a bit big. She knew about the thyroid gland because my auntie had had Graves' disease. Over the next few years my goitre became more obvious. Our family doctor said my thyroid felt quite soft and fleshy, and I hadn't got Graves' disease. He sent me to the hospital where they found I had antibodies in my blood, but my protein-bound iodine—an old test of thyroid function they don't do anymore—was normal. I felt perfectly well and the goitre didn't bother me.

At the age of 28 the goitre had become smaller but for the first time I had some discomfort in the front of my neck; it wasn't much although on a few occasions it hurt to swallow. Our doctor said my thyroid felt firmer but it was only slightly tender when he pressed it.

At the age of 48 I began to feel tired. I thought it was the change and having to look after my two teenage daughters. My periods were a bit heavier and I had to push myself to do the house work and the shopping. Eventually I went back to the doctor. He did some tests and said my thyroid was having difficulty in making hormone because my TSH was up and the thyroid hormone was down. Our GP said he couldn't feel my goitre any more but I was hypothyroid. That's when he started me on thyroxine. My periods came back and I didn't have the change until I was 54.

Few people with Hashimoto's thyroiditis will be aware of all these different stages and not many doctors may be in practice long enough to follow an individual patient over the 30–40 years involved.

Questions and Answers

*Q.*1   What exactly is an auto-immune disease?

A.   Certain defensive cells in your body which are there to fight diseases, particularly infectious diseases, have mistakenly decided that your thyroid cells are not yours—they are 'foreign' enemy cells. Auto-immune disease of the thyroid gland can cause either under- or over-activity of hormone production.

*Q.*2   Why have I got an underactive thyroid gland when my aunt had an overactive one?

A.   Both you and your aunt have auto-immune diseases. In her case her 'soldiers', which we call antibodies, stimulated her thyroid gland whereas your antibodies are killing off your thyroid cells.

*Q.*3   Will the swelling in my neck get smaller with treatment?

A.   Almost certainly, if you take your tablets regularly and go on taking them.

*Q.*4   Ought I to have my children tested to see if they are going to get an auto-immune disease?

A.   At the ages of five and three they are too young. They *may* possibly develop an auto-immune disease later in life, but it is too early to tell. In other words the tests might be negative now, only to become positive later in life. It's unlikely that they will but the best thing to do is to wait. If either of them develops a goitre, then obviously tests must be done.

8

Underactivity of the thyroid
and its causes

Causes

There are many causes for thyroid deficiency. Worldwide the commonest is probably lack of dietary iodine (p. 4). Deficiency of this essential element precludes the thyroid cells from getting enough raw material to make sufficient thyroid hormones. This is an example of trying to make bricks without straw and is usually associated with the development of a sizeable goitre. But, as we have seen in Chapter 7, Hashimoto's disease is the most usual cause of hypothyroidism in the Western world. Also a significant number of people develop hypothyroidism after radio-iodine treatment (p. 40) or surgery (p. 42) for the correction of thyroid overactivity. Usually this thyroid deficiency is permanent but sometimes, shortly after surgical or radio-iodine treatment, it may be transient.

Other less common causes of thyroid underactivity, which in some cases may be only transient or remit when the cause is removed, include:

1. Antithyroid drugs such as methimazole or carbimazole if given in too large a dose over too long a period of time will induce thyroid deficiency by impeding the manufacture of thyroid hormones by the thyroid cells.
2. Medicines purchased over the chemist's counter, particularly for coughs, may contain iodides and in some people their prolonged usage causes underactivity of the thyroid.
3. Other medicines prescribed by doctors may interfere with the function of the thyroid gland. Lithium which is used for certain mental disorders is one such, and amiodarone used for stopping irregularity of the heart beat is another.
4. Certain foods such as cabbage and other 'greens' related to kale (notably in Tasmania), seaweed (particularly in Japan) and certain so-called health foods contain antithyroid compounds as do some contaminated sources of water.

5. A congenital chemical abnormality in the thyroid gland which prevents it making T_4 and T_3 properly (p. 81).
6. Temporary underactivity of the gland which occurs in about one in ten women after childbirth (p. 101).
7. Sometimes thyroid failure occurs secondary to some disorder that stops the pituitary gland from secreting the thyroid-stimulating hormone (TSH). Usually other hormones normally formed by the pituitary are also deficient in hypopituitarism. A major finding in this situation is a low or absent level of TSH in the blood as compared with the raised level found when the problem is confined solely to the thyroid gland.

What happens if you have an underactive thyroid gland?

Hypothyroidism is the name given to the clinical condition that develops when there is inadequate secretion of thyroxine (T_4) and to a lesser extent of triiodothyronine (T_3). Irrespective of the cause of the thyroid underactivity the symptoms are in general the same, and their severity depends upon the degree of thyroid failure and upon its rate of onset. Myxoedema is the word used to describe untreated hypothyroidism of advanced degree and usually of long-standing.

Hypothyroidism should be looked upon as a graded phenomenon ranging from a slight impairment of thyroid function as shown by a rise in the TSH level and few if any symptoms, and progressing through a greater reduction of thyroid hormones with more likelihood of symptoms, to complete thyroid failure that will make you feel really ill and is often obvious to your doctor and associated with very abnormal laboratory tests (Table 3).

In most cases thyroid underactivity creeps up on you. The changes are so imperceptibly slow in their development that for some long time they are not recognized by you or those closest to you.

Overt hypothyroidism in the adult

The first thing you may notice is tiredness which gets progressively worse. You feel run-down and sluggish. You may find that you feel the cold more than those around you. You may want more domestic heating later in the spring or earlier in the autumn than others in your household. Unconsciously you may wear thicker clothes when the rest of the

Table 3   The grading of thyroid failure

Grade	Symptoms	Free T$_4$	Free T$_3$	TSH
Compensated	None	Normal	Normal	Slightly raised
Occult hypothyroidism	None or mild	Slightly low	Normal	Raised
Overt hypothyroidism	Mild or marked	Low	Low or low normal	Very raised

family are more lightly clad. Your periods may become heavier and last longer; sometimes they stop altogether. You may gain some weight but seldom more than 10 lb (4 kg) over a year. Your skin may become dry and thicker; your scalp hair may come out more than it used to. Your eyebrows may become sparse and the hair on your forearms short and stubbly. Axillary and pubic hair may become scanty. Your hands become podgy and your voice deeper in pitch. Your hearing may, unbeknown to you, become dulled so you are the last person in the house to hear the telephone bell. Your bowels are likely to be constipated (Fig. 6). Aches and cramps in the muscles are common, and in the night or on waking in the morning you may experience pins and needles in your fingers and hand. This is due to a nerve at the wrist becoming trapped (carpal tunnel syndrome)—a condition likely to improve when your thyroid deficiency is corrected.

The older person with thyroid deficiency may experience a tight constricting pain across the chest when walking fast or up an incline— pain which causes you to stop walking for a while until the tightness wears off. This is called angina pectoris and is due to narrowing of the coronary arteries that carry blood to your heart. Similarly if the arteries to your legs are furred up, you may experience pain in one or other calf when you walk, and this too will cause you to stop until the pain wears off (intermittent claudication).

In advanced cases of myxoedema the patient feels unsteady on her feet and once she has fallen she may be reluctant to venture out of the house alone. Words are less clearly articulated so that speech is slowed and slurred. Rarely in severe untreated cases the myxoedematous patient

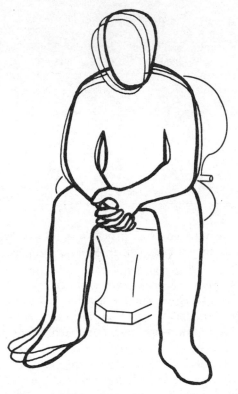

Fig. 6 A representation of a patient with thyroid deficiency (hypothyroidism).
The hypothyroid patient is slowed down, physically and mentally, and is likely to
be constipated as implied in this drawing. Compare with the hyperthyroid patient
shown in Fig. 4 (p. 32).

may become mentally disturbed. She may hear voices, believe her food is
being poisoned, and become agitated. This is all likely to get better
gradually as the thyroid deficiency is corrected. Because their metabolism
is so slow, some patients may become unconscious, particularly during
cold weather (myxoedema coma). This tends to happen in older women
who live alone and are not visited by friends or relatives. Myxoedema
coma is a serious condition and often ends fatally.

Mild hypothyroidism

If you have a minor degree of thyroid deficiency your symptoms will be more vague. Tiredness for which you can think of no physical or emotional reason, lack of 'go', intolerance of cold, dryness of your skin, constipation, heavy periods, and a feeling of bloatedness may all occur.

What your doctor finds

Depending on the degree of thyroid deficiency the changes in you may or may not be obvious to your doctor. If the underactivity is marked and if the doctor knows you well and has not seen you for some months, he may immediately suspect what is wrong with you. He may find that your face has become puffy. Your skin may have a yellow tinge although your cheeks may remain surprisingly pink unless your heavy periods have made you anaemic. He or she may spot that your eyelids and hands are puffy, sometimes with swelling of the ankles. Your movements, your speech and thoughts may be slowed. Your heart rate is likely to be slow, and your blood pressure somewhat elevated. Your tendon reflexes are slow to relax (p. 20). Sometimes fluid will have collected in your abdomen, in your chest or in the envelope that surrounds your heart so that you become short of breath.

If the cause of your hypothyroidism is Hashimoto's disease, your thyroid gland may be slightly enlarged, normal in size, or so destroyed that your doctor cannot feel it. If the gland can be felt, it will be harder than normal. Sometimes your doctor may find one or two nodules in it which are usually small areas of normal thyroid tissue that have escaped the auto-immune inflammatory attack but are insufficient in amount to sustain normal thyroid function.

Diagnosis of adult hypothyroidism

The abnormalities in the thyroid function tests depend on the severity of the deficiency (Table 3). In clinically obvious hypothyroidism, the T_4 and to a lesser extent the T_3 level are depressed below the normal range and the TSH level is very high. In milder cases only the T_4 level is low normal or below normal with a raised TSH level.

Certain indirect tests for detecting thyroid deficiency or for following its response to treatment have been used. The sluggishness of the tendon reflexes may be measured (p. 20). The blood cholesterol is often raised in thyroid deficiency and comes down in response to adequate treatment.

The electrocardiogram may show changes which disappear with treatment.

Your doctor is likely to look for thyroid antibodies unless he already knows that you have Hashimoto's disease or the cause for your thyroid deficiency is obvious because you have had thyroid surgery or been treated with radio-iodine. The finding of antibodies raises the possibility that you may be prone, sooner or later, to some other auto-immune disease (p. 112 *et seq.*).

If your doctor does not know you well a comparison of your present appearance with an earlier photograph may be helpful in suggesting a diagnosis of hypothyroidism. Pictures taken before and after replacement treatment with thyroxine are often a witness to the striking therapeutic response (Plate 15).

Thyroid underactivity in children

The onset of thyroid underfunction in children around the age of 8 is usually due to imperfect development or maldescent (p. 2) of the thyroid gland earlier in life, or to Hashimoto's thyroiditis. Less often the cause is some congenital defect whereby the manufacture of T_4 and T_3 by the thyroid cells is impaired (dyshormonogenesis).

When the gland has not developed properly the amount of thyroid tissue may have been adequate initially to sustain normal levels of the thyroid hormones, but as the child grows the maldeveloped gland cannot keep pace and thyroid deficiency gradually develops.

The most obvious consequence of thyroid underactivity at this age is that the child stops growing. Seldom are there other symptoms and surprisingly the child's performance at school is usually maintained. Although failure to grow is the presenting feature, the child is often plump and may have pads of fat above the collar-bones. Sexual development and puberty may be delayed but in some long-standing cases sexual development is unduly advanced.

The diagnosis is based on the same tests as are used for confirming thyroid underactivity in the adult. In addition X-rays will show that the development of the bones is delayed in relation to the child's chronological age. An isotope scan of the neck will show the gland is abnormally small in maldevelopment, and in maldescent (p. 23) the uptake will be near the root of the tongue instead of in the normal position.

Thyroid underactivity in the new-born

Thyroid failure in the new-born, if unrecognized, can be disastrous because delay in treatment results in permanent mental deficiency (cretinism). In the Western world the most common cause of congenital hypothyroidism is maldevelopment or maldescent of the thyroid gland. The prevalence is 30 to 40 cases per 100 000 births. Thus in developed countries every new-born baby is screened to exclude thyroid deficiency.

In areas of the world where iodine deficiency is common (p. 4) the prevalence of neonatal hypothyroidism is high and the degree of mental defect and damage to the nervous system is great. In these cases the baby's mother usually has a goitre caused by lack of iodine and possibly to other antithyroid factors in her diet or drinking water. This type of endemic neonatal hypothyroidism can be prevented by giving the mother injections of iodized oil or fortifying her salt or bread with iodides.

What does a baby with thyroid deficiency look like?

The answer is that in many cases the baby looks perfectly normal even to the trained experienced eye. That is why in so-called developed countries a screening test is done routinely on every new-born baby. When there are abnormal features, these depend upon the degree of thyroid deficiency and become more obvious as the baby grows older, but by then permanent damage to the brain may have occurred. Babies with thyroid deficiency fail to thrive. The baby does not kick vigorously and sleeps excessively. Constipation is the rule. The baby's cry may be croaky. The scalp hair may be short and coarse. Often the tummy is unduly protuberant; the navel may bulge outwards and be the site of a rupture. The tongue is unusually large and to the experienced eye the face may have a characteristic flat bloated look. Left untreated changes due to involvement of the brain appear—poor co-ordination, shakiness, and unsteadiness with excessively brisk tendon reflexes.

Without doing a screening test many babies with neonatal thyroid deficiency are not diagnosed until they are 6 months old and cretinism is then irreversible. Although the physical changes will disappear with thyroxine treatment, the mental state is likely to remain permanently impaired.

Diagnosis of neonatal hypothyroidism

Every new-born baby should be screened for thyroid deficiency on the fifth to tenth day after birth. A needle prick will be made in your baby's heel and four spots of blood are placed on a special piece of paper. Two of these spots are analysed for TSH and the other two are used to screen for another congenital disease (phenylketonuria). In babies with thyroid deficiency the TSH is substantially raised. When the level is not all that high, the test has to be repeated. Sometimes congenital thyroid deficiency is transient, and without treatment your baby would develop normal thyroid function. This is liable to happen in premature births and in babies of mothers who have been taking thyroid hormone, antithyroid drugs, or iodine-containing drugs during the pregnancy. It is safer to treat all infants with a positive test and when your baby is about a year old to stop the replacement treatment for a few weeks and carefully observe the T_4 and TSH levels. If the T_4 falls and the TSH rises, thyroxine can be restarted and your infant will not suffer any permanent damage from being temporarily deprived of the replacement treatment.

Treatment

The best treatment for thyroid deficiency is replacement therapy with thyroxine. Although man-made, medicinal thyroxine is chemically identical to the natural hormone secreted by the thyroid gland. Being a pure substance the amount in each tablet made by a reputable pharmaceutical company is precise and accurate. Two strengths of tablet are widely available throughout the world—0.05 milligrams (mg), also expressed as 50 micrograms (μg or mcg), and 0.1 mg (100 μg or mcg). In some countries, such as the UK and North America, tablets of 0.025 mg (25 μg or mcg) are also available, and in others such as the United States additional strengths are made. Thyroxine is a stable substance and the tablets have a long shelf-life.

The starting or initial dose of thyroxine you will be given will depend upon:

1. Your age. Elderly people are usually started on a small dose, such as 0.025 mg so as not to upset the heart. This will certainly be necessary if you already have some heart trouble (see below).
2. The duration of time you have been thyroid deficient. If your under-activity has only just occurred as a result, say, of a thyroid operation, replacement with a larger initial dose, such as 0.1 or 0.15 mg is safe. If the deficiency is of longer standing the initial dose may be 0.05 mg.

The dosage of thyroxine will be adjusted by your doctor according to how you feel and the results of laboratory tests. Adjustment of the dosage is unlikely to be made more often than at intervals of 2–8 weeks. There is a good deal of debate among thyroid experts about what the aim, as regards the results of the laboratory tests, should be. Every one agrees that enough thyroxine should be given to bring the TSH level down into the normal range. This may result in the serum total or free T_4 level being above the normal range but this does not seem to matter as long as the total or free T_3 level is in the normal range. The ultimate dose of thyroxine you need will depend upon your degree of thyroid failure and your age. The total daily dose in an adult with no functioning thyroid tissue at all is usually 0.15–0.2 mg. Occasionally the dose may need to be 0.25 mg.

Thyroxine does not work quickly. A tablet taken, for example, on a Monday will induce no biologically discernible effect in your body until the next Friday. Thus you need take your tablets only once a day. There is no point in taking them two or three times a day; indeed there may be a positive disadvantage in doing so because you are likely to forget a dose, particularly the midday one. Thus take your tablets once a day at a time when you will not forget—perhaps when you brush your teeth in the morning before breakfast.

Do not expect to feel miraculously better overnight. The longer you have had thyroid deficiency the longer it will take for you to feel really well again—sometimes as long as 6–9 months. It takes this length of time for the changes in your tissues to be reversed.

Initial problems

Elderly patients, even with a small starting dose of thyroxine, may develop heart problems, such as palpitations, irregularity of the pulse, shortness of breath, ankle swelling or angina. Some younger people experience intermittent and innocent palpitations when they start treatment. A small dose of a beta-blocker, such as 10–20 mg propranolol twice or three times daily, will usually quell these symptoms.

Some people, particularly the older ones with long-standing thyroid deficiency, may during the early phases of replacement treatment experience the 'screws'—muscular aches and pains particularly in the thighs, arms, and back. Do not stop your medication if this happens to you. A simple pain-killing medicine will help make you feel more comfortable until this problem has passed.

After you have been stabilized, it is sensible to ask your doctor for a signed document setting forth how your thyroid deficiency came to light, the results of the tests that confirmed it, and your current replacement dosage of thyroxine. This may be useful if in the years to come you change doctors or go to live abroad. Your new doctor, who finds you well, may doubt the need for continued treatment and stop the thyroxine.

Your replacement dosage of thyroxine may need adjustment as you grow older. If you have Hashimoto's disease your degree of thyroid deficiency may increase and necessitate an increased dose of thyroxine. As you get even older you may require a smaller dose. For these reasons your thyroid status should ideally be checked every 1 or 2 years.

Some people with thyroid deficiency take too much thyroxine in the mistaken hope that it will help them to lose weight and because they feel 'better' with a thyroxine level in the blood raised far above the upper normal range. There is no doubt that some people do get 'addicted' to thyroxine and take doses that make them hyperthyroid. This has an adverse effect on the heart and also induces thinning of the bones (osteoporosis) with an enhanced liability for you to break your hip, wrist, or the bones in your spine.

Other drugs have been used for the treatment of thyroid deficiency but have little to commend them. Thyroid extract is prepared from the dried thyroid glands of animals. It is an impure substance of variable biological potency with a short shelf-life. It is no longer listed in the British National Formulary.

Triiodothyronine (T_3) is sometimes used but it has no advantage over thyroxine except in the treatment of myxoedema coma. Triiodothyronine has a quick, short duration of action and the tablets should not be taken in a single daily dose. If T_3 is used the correct dosage cannot be judged by the blood level of total T_4 or free T_4 (both of which will be suppressed) but by the TSH and the total or free T_3 levels.

Treatment of thyroid deficiency in babies and children follows the same pattern as that in grown-ups. The initial dose of thyroxine for a baby is 0.025 mg every day or every other day, and for children 0.05 mg daily. The dosage will have to be increased as they grow older and is best judged by the blood T_3 and TSH levels. Additional assessment of the response is made from the child's growth in height and from the maturing of the bones as judged by simple X-rays of the hand and wrist. A child given too much thyroxine is likely to become overactive, unduly excitable and will grow faster than normal.

Questions and Answers

Q.1   I've taken the tablets prescribed for me a month ago, but I can't say I'm feeling any better.

A.   It's taken months, perhaps years, for you to develop thyroid underactivity and it may take 4 months or more before you are completely well again.

Q.2   My son was diagnosed as having thyroid deficiency in hospital, just after he was born. Now he's a year old, and the hospital want to stop the thyroxine for the next month and then do another test. Is that safe?

A.   Yes it's safe; and it's the only way to find out if he really needs the thyroxine now.

Q.3   I have been on thyroxine treatment for two months and my period was very heavy again last month. Is this going to get better?

A.   Almost certainly. It takes time for everything to return to normal.

Q.4   Does it matter when I take my thyroid tablets?

A.   No, you can take them at any time of the day provided you always remember to take them. Most people are less likely to forget if they take them first thing in the morning when they brush their teeth.

Q.5   The tablets I got this month from the chemist are larger than the previous ones I had. The old ones were labelled 0.1 mg thyroxine but the new ones are 100 micrograms. Hasn't the chemist made a mistake? I feel all right.

A.   0.1 milligrams is the same as 100 micrograms. Several different reputable manufacturers make thyroxine tablets and the different makes are not all the same size, although they may contain exactly the same amount of the hormone. However, there are different strengths of thyroxine tablets, and you are right to check that you are taking the correct dose.

9

Subacute viral thyroiditis

This condition, also known as de Quervain's thyroiditis after the Swiss physician who first described it, appears to be particularly common in North America. This may be because familiarity with the disease results in the diagnosis being made more often there. Because viral thyroiditis runs a self-limiting course, mild cases may never seek medical advice and there can be no doubt that even in more severe cases the correct diagnosis is often overlooked.

The condition occurs more commonly in women than men and those with a pre-existing small goitre seem more vulnerable. The inflammation of the thyroid is caused by one of several viruses. The most common is the Coxsackie virus (first isolated in a small township of that name in New York State) but the mumps virus and others may be the cause. Attempts are seldom made to identify the causative virus in any particular patient because the technique to do so is expensive and difficult, and we do not yet have many generally effective antiviral agents.

What is subacute viral thyroiditis like?

The disease varies from very mild to quite severe. One of your authors (R.I.S.B.), having had mild de Quervain's thyroiditis himself, is in a good position to tell you, so forgive him for being personal!

One summer's day, when I was aged 45, I felt exceptionally and unreasonably tired. I went to bed immediately after supper and feeling hot I took my temperature. I had a slight fever of 37.7 °C (99 °F). I slept all right but next morning woke with a generalised headache and ached all over. My temperature was only marginally raised so I went to work. Again I went to bed early and the headache was bad enough for me to take an aspirin. I reckoned I'd got 'flu. The next few days were much the same. After a week of coming home early and going to bed, my wife reminded me that a professor of endocrinology from out of town was coming to dine with us. He was an old friend so I came down to supper in my dressing gown, and told him I was getting over a brief attack of 'flu.

After dinner my professor friend said, 'Are you sure you haven't got thyroiditis?'

'I shouldn't think so,' I said. 'Why do you ask?'

'Because you've gently been rubbing your neck all evening as though it hurt.'

'Well, now you mention it, it does.' I prodded my thyroid gland. 'Yes, it's quite tender and it hurts a bit when I swallow too. What's more I get stabs of pain that run up the side of my neck to just under my ears.'

The next day I was worse and asked our family doctor, who lives close by and was a good friend, to look in. He took my history and examined me from top to toe. (I did not mention thyroiditis because doctors who make a self-diagnosis can also make fools of themselves!) The G.P. looked puzzled. 'I'll drop in early tomorrow,' he said, 'and take some blood off you.'

Next morning he said, 'Would you think I'm mad if I said I thought you'd got subacute viral thyroiditis? I've read the chapter you write about de Quervain's disease in that large Oxford text book of medicine you contribute to. It seems to me you're a classic mild case.'

He was right, but as you will see there was more to come.

So if you get subacute viral thyroiditis, the illness usually starts with a generalized 'flu-like illness with tiredness, muscular aches and pains, a mild headache, and a slight fever. After a few days the virus concentrates on your thyroid gland which becomes slightly enlarged, painful, and tender. Swallowing hurts and characteristically stabs of pain run up the front of your neck to the ear on one or both sides.

Because the gland is inflamed by the virus, the pre-formed thyroid hormones leach out into the bloodstream and the levels of thyroid hormones rise. This induces the symptoms of hyperthyroidism and you become mildly thyrotoxic.

I certainly could feel my heart beating away at 80–90 a minute even when I was resting in bed; I was sweaty and irritable. I ate well enough but lost 4 lbs (1.8 kg) in the second week and rather less the next. My hands became shaky when holding a teacup. It took me about a month to get over it, and all I took was some aspirin.

You may go to your doctor complaining, perfectly rightly, of a sore throat. Unless *you* make it clear you mean the soreness is in the front of your neck, your doctor may focus his attention on the throat at the back of your mouth and find that the tonsillar area is normal or slightly pinker than normal. Unless he perceives that it is your thyroid gland in your neck that is sore, the diagnosis may well be missed.

Most people with subacute viral thyroiditis get well in 3–6 weeks, and a stoical patient may ignore the symptoms altogether. If you have a worse attack you will be ill for rather longer, with symptoms that wax and wane, and you may feel quite ill for a time.

How is the diagnosis confirmed?

Provided the diagnosis is suspected from your history and what your doctor finds, it can easily be confirmed. During the acute inflammatory phase the blood levels of T_4 and T_3 are raised and because of the feedback mechanism your TSH is suppressed. The way to distinguish this from other causes of thyroid overactivity is to do an isotope scan. Because the thyroid cells are so deranged by the inflammation caused by the virus, they do not take up the isotope. With reference to the analogy of the car factory in Chapter 3 (p. 19), this is a situation when no raw steel is going into the factory yet more than the normal number of finished cars are coming out at the other end.

Sometimes it is necessary for your doctor to distinguish subacute viral thyroiditis from the early stages of Hashimoto's thyroiditis (Chapter 7) when there may be some discomfort in the thyroid produced by the auto-immune inflammation associated with mildly increased hormone secretion (Hashitoxicosis, p. 59). In this condition the uptake of isotope is normal or increased, not zero as in viral thyroiditis, and the key to the diagnosis is also the high level of thyroid auto-antibodies in Hashimoto's disease. The tenderness of the thyroid in subacute viral thyroiditis distinguishes the condition from Graves' disease.

Treatment

If you have mild de Quervain's disease you may need no treatment beyond aspirin or paracetamol (acetaminophen) to relieve the discomfort in your neck. If the symptoms of thyrotoxicosis are troublesome, treatment with a beta-blocker is usually adequate to control them. If the discomfort in your neck is not controlled by simple analgesics, prednisone or prednisolone (cortisone-like drugs) reduces the inflammation in your thyroid gland. Initially you will probably be given a fairly large dose (30–40 mg daily) for the first week and then the amount is gradually reduced over the next 3 weeks. Some people experience a relapse and the course of steroids has to be repeated.

It is unusual for the thyroid gland to be damaged permanently although after the acute phase you may for a time have temporary thyroid deficiency.

Questions and Answers

*Q.*1 The tablets I was prescribed a week ago have helped: I'm in much less of a state and my heart is not banging around, but my neck still hurts a lot. In fact I think it's more painful than it was and swallowing hurts. Can anything else be done?

A. The beta-blocker, the propranolol, is obviously helping. That's why your heart is quieter and you're not so het up. However, the paracetamol (acetaminophen) is obviously not strong enough to relieve your pain, and it may be advisable for you to take some prednisone for 4-8 weeks instead.

*Q.*2 Is this thyroid trouble going to cause permanent damage?

A. Almost certainly not. Most people get over subacute viral thyroiditis without permanent damage. There is a very faint chance that your thyroid gland might become underactive, but in that case the deficiency can easily be corrected.

*Q.*3 Why have I got this disease?

A. It is caused by a virus, but it is rarely possible to find out which one. Occasionally it is due to the mumps virus but so far there is no treatment that is effective against this sort of virus.

*Q.*4 My wife or the children won't catch this disease from me, will they?

A. No.

10

Uniform enlargement of the thyroid and simple non-toxic goitre

The word 'goitre' simply means enlargement of your thyroid gland. It may not always be easy for your doctor to decide whether or not your thyroid is enlarged unless you have an obvious goitre because the normal thyroid gland varies in size from person to person, and it varies in different parts of the world, being larger in areas where there is iodine deficiency. In young women with a long thin neck the thyroid may just be visible, particularly if you hold your chin up, but in most normal people the thyroid is not visible. A small goitre is defined as one that your doctor can feel to be larger than normal even though the gland may not be visible. However in most instances an obvious goitre is visible and it certainly feels larger than normal.

Do not be unduly alarmed if you develop slight generalized enlargement of your thyroid gland. It is most unlikely that you have cancer, because cancer of the thyroid is a rare condition. Furthermore, cancer of the thyroid seldom causes a generalized uniform enlargement.

Some enlargement of the thyroid is quite common. In a survey done in the north-east of England a few years ago nearly 16 per cent of the population had small or obvious goitres, with a female to male ratio of 4 to 1 which emphasizes how much more common thyroid enlargement is in women than in men.

In this chapter we discuss enlargement of the thyroid gland in which the enlargement is uniform and more or less involves the whole gland equally. In Chapter 11 we will discuss enlargement of the thyroid gland that is due to the development of lumps or nodules in it. This division into uniform and nodular enlargement is somewhat artificial because often the two occur together but the distinction is helpful in working out why you have a goitre.

There are many causes for uniform enlargement of the thyroid and in the Western world, where there is little iodine deficiency, the most common cause is what is called a *simple non-toxic goitre*, which will be discussed at the end of this chapter. First let us look at some of the other causes of a uniform goitre.

Causes of a uniform goitre

'Normal' or physiological causes

Slight enlargement of the thyroid gland is common in girls at or soon after the onset of puberty, and quite a number of normal women notice that their thyroid gland becomes slightly larger during the 7-10 days before their menstrual period.

Enlargement of the gland is also common in pregnancy. In ancient Egypt it was the practice to tie a thin thread tightly round the neck of a young bride. When the thread broke it was evidence that she had become pregnant. Hormonal changes are probably responsible for your thyroid becoming larger under these circumstances but it has also been suggested that a minor degree of iodine deficiency may sometimes be a factor, particularly in pregnancy. When you are pregnant, the baby growing inside you needs iodine and you lose more iodine in your urine. Hence your body stores of iodine may become somewhat reduced.

At the time of the menopause slight enlargement of the thyroid may also occur.

Iodine deficiency and endemic goitre

Worldwide this is the commonest cause of a goitre, but it only occurs in areas where there is lack of iodine in the diet and/or the diet contains antithyroid or goitre-producing substances that interfere with the manufacture of the thyroid hormones. Iodine is essential for the manufacture of the thyroid hormones, and if iodine is in short supply the thyroid gland may enlarge under the influence of the thyroid-stimulating hormone secreted by the pituitary in an attempt, sometimes successful, to maintain a normal level of thyroid hormones in the bloodstream. The iodine content of food, contained mainly in milk, eggs, and vegetables, largely depends upon the amount of iodine in the soil and this in turn depends upon the fall of rain derived from sea-water. Thus iodine deficiency is found in areas far removed from the sea. Such was the case in Alpine countries such as Switzerland, around the Great Lakes in the United States and even in the Pennines in England ('Derbyshire neck') until corrective measures were taken to fortify salt and bread with iodine.

However iodine deficiency is still common in large land-locked areas such as the Himalayas, parts of China, Iran, the Congo basin, the Andes, and in New Guinea where preventive measures are still imperfect. In these parts of the world goitre is so common that it affects 20 per cent or more of the population and is therefore called endemic.

In iodine-deficient regions there is a direct relationship between the degree of iodine deficiency and the prevalence of goitre. If the deficiency is marked, and this can be assessed by finding only very small amounts of iodine in a 24-hour urine collection, a large proportion of the population will have a goitre. In certain isolated areas such as New Guinea the incidence of goitre and the risk of an iodine-deficient goitrous mother giving birth to a baby with thyroid deficiency has been reduced by giving the mother every five years an injection of iodized poppy-seed oil.

Hashimoto's disease

As a cause of goitre this is discussed in Chapter 7. In areas where there is little deficiency of iodine as in the Western world it is a common cause of thyroid enlargement, which may be present long before underactivity of the gland develops. That this chronic lymphocytic thyroiditis is the cause of a goitre is confirmed by finding thyroid auto-antibodies in your blood, and this helps to distinguish Hashimoto's disease from simple non-toxic goitre (see below).

Graves' disease

As explained in Chapter 4 this is a cause of goitre. If you develop thyroid enlargement because you have thyrotoxicosis, you will be more concerned by the symptoms produced by the thyroid overactivity than by the usually modest enlargement of your thyroid gland.

Subacute viral thyroiditis

As a cause of goitre this is discussed in Chapter 9, but this condition is unlikely to be confused with simple non-toxic goitre because your thyroid gland will hurt and be tender to the touch.

Foods and drugs

Certain foods and drugs, some recognized and some not, interfere with the manufacture of thyroid hormones. Cabbage, certain vegetables of the kale family, and cassava, which is consumed as a staple diet in Africa, may produce a goitre when eaten in large quantities or when milk is drunk from cows that have been fed on kale. Similarly certain medicines from your chemist, notably cough and asthma cures, may cause thyroid enlargement when taken over a long period of time. Many drugs, ranging from those used for the treatment of irregularities of the heart beat to those used to treat certain mental illnesses may cause the thyroid to enlarge. If you develop a goitre you must tell your doctor about all the drugs, medicines, or herbal remedies that you are taking or have taken during previous months.

Disturbed manufacture of thyroid hormones

The making of your thyroid hormones involves many orderly chemical steps and normally each is precisely regulated in the same way as the assembly of a motorcar involves many distinct stages. In some people the synthesis of thyroid hormones may be slowed down at one particular stage. This is called dyshormonogenesis, a long word that means literally 'disordered genesis (formation) of hormones'. The severity of the disorder may vary from a very mild hiccup in the synthetic process to a more major hold-up.

Goitres caused by dyshormonogenesis are very rare and tend to run in families. Usually the condition declares itself soon after birth because the baby has a goitre. In others the abnormality does not become noticeable until some years later because, as the child grows and the need for thyroid hormone increases, the gland enlarges in an attempt to meet the demand. In rare instances disordered thyroid hormone synthesis is associated with other congenital problems, such as deafness.

In most instances treatment with thyroxine prevents the goitre from getting any larger and often makes it smaller. Furthermore such treatment obviates the risk of the patient becoming thyroid hormone deficient.

Cancer

As a cause of goitre cancer is discussed in Chapter 12. However in malignant thyroid disease the enlargement of the thyroid gland is seldom uniform and is much more likely to be nodular.

Simple non-toxic goitre

The adjectives 'simple non-toxic' mean that the goitre is not cancerous and it is unassociated with any abnormality of thyroid secretory function. In other words if you develop a simple non-toxic goitre, you will be euthyroid. 'Simple' does not imply that the mechanism causing the enlargement is easily explained; indeed the cause of a simple non-toxic goitre, also sometimes known as a *colloid goitre* or a *simple goitre*, is not really known.

How do you feel?

Most people with a small non-toxic goitre are unaware of its presence and they have no symptoms. Understandably you may become apprehensive if you see in the mirror that your thyroid gland is enlarged, or a relative tells you that it is. A few people immediately complain of 'a lump in the throat', difficulty in swallowing, or a choking feeling. Because quite large goitres seldom cause any symptoms at all, it is likely that any symptoms in those with a small goitre are more the consequences of apprehension than related to the enlargement of the thyroid gland.

In many instances the investigation of someone with a simple non-toxic goitre is as important in allaying their fears as it is in determining the cause of the thyroid enlargement and how best to treat it.

What your doctor finds

Initially a simple non-toxic goitre is not large although it may be obvious. It is symmetrical, and feels smooth and soft. It is painless. If whatever is causing the goitre persists or the condition is left untreated, the goitre may become, as the years pass, more irregular and contain several nodules (a multinodular goitre), or one part of the gland becomes more prominent than another (see Chapter 11).

Complications

Any complications from a simple non-toxic goitre are unusual except in neglected cases.

Pressure symptoms.   Left untreated a simple goitre may, rarely, grow to sufficient size to cause pressure symptoms by virtue of its bulk. The large veins in the neck bringing blood back to the heart from the head may become compressed. The veins then stand out on one or both sides of your neck, and you may have a sense of fullness in the face with the development of swelling below the eyes and facial puffiness.

The windpipe may be compressed if the goitre becomes very large, especially if part of the goitre lies behind the breast-bone (p. 1). The windpipe may be pushed to one side and compressed if your thyroid is asymmetrically enlarged. In extreme cases breathing is partially obstructed and when asleep you may make a curious crowing noise (stridor).

Involvement of the nerves to the vocal cords. Very seldom indeed does pressure from a non-malignant goitre impair the function of the nerves that activate the vocal cords. If you develop weakness or hoarseness of your voice you should see your doctor forthwith.

Hypothyroidism. Over the years a simple goitre may fail to produce sufficient thyroid hormones, either because the initial cause for the goitre persists or because the gland becomes involved, as a separate entity, by Hashimoto's auto-immune disease (Chapter 7).

Hyperthyroidism. Sometimes thyroid overactivity develops in a simple non-toxic goitre that has progressed to a multinodular goitre (p. 86). If this happens an isotope scan is likely to show increased activity in the tissue between the nodules and it is thought that you have developed a second thyroid disorder, namely Graves' disease (Chapter 4).

Diagnosis of simple non-toxic goitre

Although a careful history is taken and extensive tests may be done, it is often impossible to discover the cause of a simple non-toxic goitre. Thyroid function tests (the blood levels of T_4, T_3, and TSH) are normal. There is nothing to suggest iodine deficiency, no evidence of auto-immune thyroid disease (i.e. no thyroid auto-antibodies) and no clear evidence of abnormal thyroid hormone manufacture. As you will now understand, the diagnosis of simple non-toxic goitre is based on proving a lot of negatives, although the condition may run in families which suggests a mild form of dyshormonogenesis. Nor is there any history of eating peculiar foods or taking drugs that may induce a goitre. In the early stages an isotope scan will show a normal pattern of uptake.

Treatment

The logical approach to treatment of a simple non-toxic goitre would be to correct or remove the cause, but as this is unknown this is not possible. However, on the assumption that most cases are related either to slight, perhaps intermittent, iodine lack or to a minor degree of dyshormonogenesis or to both, control of the goitre is possible.

First a normal dietary intake of iodine must be assured and any deficiency or excess (Kelp, seaweed, medicines, or drugs) avoided. Iodized salt or sea salt are widely available and clearly labelled as 'iodized'. This type of salt should be used in cooking and at the table. Sea fish is a good source of iodine.

If your goitre is small, an adequate intake of iodine may be all that is required to prevent your thyroid from growing larger and may make the goitre smaller. It is sensible for you to remain under regular observation, initially every 4 months and later every year for a few years. In many patients nothing more is required.

If your gland increases in size with an adequate iodine intake—and this means neither too little nor too much—or your gland is already large when you first seek medical advice, treatment with thyroxine is used. The initial dose is usually 0.05 mg daily but this may be increased to 0.1 mg or 0.15 mg daily. In patients aged 15–30 this treatment is usually continued for about 3 years and then reduced and finally stopped. A careful watch is kept on the size of your goitre. In some people the position remains static but in others the thyroid begins to enlarge again and lifelong thyroxine treatment then becomes necessary with regular supervision.

In those who do not seek advice until the thyroid is so large that it is cosmetically unsightly or it has become a multinodular goitre surgery may have to be considered. Subtotal thyroidectomy may particularly be indicated if your sizeable goitre is causing compression symptoms or if the gland lies behind the breast-bone. After the operation it will be necessary for you to take thyroxine for the rest of your life to prevent the remaining thyroid tissue from increasing in size.

Questions and Answers

Q.   What do you mean exactly when you say I've got a goitre?

A.   The word goitre simply means enlargement of your thyroid gland.

Q.2 Does it mean that I've got cancer?

A.   Certainly not. Most goitres are *not* malignant.

Q.3 Why have I got a goitre?

A.   I don't know—yet. That is what I am going to try to find out. There are many different causes.

Q.4 Will it get any bigger? It's ugly enough as it is!

A.   Ugly? You can't say that! Most people wouldn't notice anything wrong with you. There's a good chance that we can prevent it getting any bigger and probably we'll make it smaller.

11

Irregular enlargement of the thyroid and benign nodules

Sometimes one or more lumps may develop in your thyroid gland. Although this may happen whether your thyroid is of normal size or you already have a goitre, nodules are more likely to develop in women who already have a goitre (often of long-standing), and particularly in those who have Hashimoto's disease or a family history of thyroid disease.

In fact nodules are quite common and some may be too small for you to notice them or for your doctor to be able to feel them. The great majority are harmless.

Non-malignant lumps seldom increase suddenly in size unless bleeding into them occurs (see below); they are unattached to the overlying skin and are not associated with enlargement of the lymph glands in your neck.

Irregular enlargement of the thyroid often occurs in thyroid cancer but may also occur in Hashimoto's disease and other benign conditions.

A solitary nodule

You may develop a single nodule in your thyroid gland, or what may seem to you and your doctor to be a single nodule, but an ultrasound scan often shows that in fact you have several nodules, many of which are too small to be felt. Hence what appears to your doctor to be a solitary nodule may in fact be the visible expression of a multinodular goitre (see below and p. 82).

A solitary nodule usually appears as a smooth rounded lump that is not painful. It may contain fluid and therefore is a cyst but this can only be diagnosed with certainty from an ultrasound scan and/or by doing a needle biopsy when fluid will be withdrawn. Very few small cysts are malignant.

Sudden painful enlargement of a lump may occur if bleeding takes place into it. This happens for no known reason: the smooth round swelling increases in size over a few hours, becomes hard because of the increased pressure inside it and is painful. If a needle biopsy is done (p. 25) blood-stained fluid is withdrawn; the lump becomes less tense and the pain is relieved.

A single nodule is usually a benign non-toxic cluster of cells—benign because it is not cancerous, and non-toxic because it does not produce an excess of thyroid hormones. However a benign non-toxic nodule may, in the years ahead, produce excess thyroid hormones and make you thyrotoxic. This is discussed in Chapter 6 (p. 53).

It is always necessary to establish that your nodule is non-toxic (by doing tests of thyroid function) and that it is not malignant. This distinction between benign and cancerous is not easy and three procedures, none of which are always absolutely reliable, are used to try to make it:

1. A needle biopsy (p. 25) which may not always produce enough tissue or the appearance of the cells under the microscope may not allow the certain exclusion of cancer.
2. An ultrasound scan (p. 25) will show whether the nodule is filled with fluid and is therefore cystic, which is more likely to be benign, or solid or semi-solid which does not help distinguish between benign and malignant, a distinction that cannot be made by this technique.
3. An isotope scan (p. 23), either with radio-iodine or technetium but the former is usually preferred, which may show some uptake in a benign nodule but usually little or no uptake in a cancerous nodule. Certainly a 'cold' nodule, which does not take up the isotope, is more suspicious of cancer than a 'warm' or 'hot' one that does, but many benign lumps and cysts are also 'cold' and only about 10 per cent of 'cold' nodules turn out to be cancerous. If the isotope scan shows that in fact you have several nodules, this makes it even more unlikely that you have cancer. Furthermore it must be emphasized that benign swellings are much more common than thyroid cancer.

Because these tests for distinguishing between a benign isolated swelling and a cancerous one may not be conclusive, do not be upset if your doctor advises surgical removal of the lump. Not only will this establish the diagnosis with certainty but simple removal of the lump and some of its surrounding tissue will probably get rid of your problem.

Multiple nodules

Cancer is even less likely when the thyroid gland contains several nodules, whether or not these can be felt by your doctor or are only discovered by a scan.

Treatment

Once any question of cancer has been excluded, there may be no need for any special treatment although it would be wise for you to remain under medical surveillance. In some instances your doctor may wish to give you thyroxine because such treatment may prevent further enlargement of the nodule and may reduce the likelihood of other nodules developing. If a solitary nodule becomes overactive, treatment with radio-iodine is often used in preference to surgical removal with equally good results (p. 53). If a multinodular goitre causes thyroid overactivity, radio-iodine or surgery may be used (p. 52).

Questions and Answers

Q. 1   Is this little lump that has developed in my neck likely to be cancer?

A.   The lump is in your thyroid gland and isn't an enlarged lymph gland. It's unlikely to be malignant but tests must be done to be sure.

Q. 2   Are these tests conclusive?

A.   Not always. If there is any doubt, particularly after the biopsy, then it would be advisable to have the lump removed by a surgeon. About half the patients with a solitary nodule have to undergo surgery.

Q. 3   This lump in my neck has suddenly blown up and is really painful. What is it?

A.   You have a nodule in your thyroid gland and bleeding into it has occurred. That's why it's suddenly enlarged and become painful. If the fluid is removed from the nodule it will relieve your pain and the nodule will become less tense. Later your doctor will carry out a number of tests to find out why you've developed a nodule.

*Q.*4   My lump has disappeared since the fluid was removed from it. I was told it was a thyroid cyst. Will it come back again?

A.   It may, but if it does come back, there's a good chance that the fluid can be removed again or that you can have the cyst removed if it continues to bother you.

12

Cancer of the thyroid gland

Compared with the incidence of malignant disease elsewhere in the body, cancer of the thyroid gland is rare and is responsible for less than 0.5 per cent of all deaths from cancer. Only 6 people per million of the population die of the disease each year in England and Wales. Although it may occur at any age, it is most common between the ages of 30 and 60, and as with other thyroid disorders it is more common in women.

What is the cause of thyroid cancer?

Although the precise cause of thyroid cancer is unknown, previous X-ray treatment to the head, neck, or chest is certainly a predisposing factor. There was a vogue before World War II and in the 1940s, particularly in certain centres in the United States, to reduce the size of enlarged tonsils and adenoids in children by X-ray therapy in preference to surgical removal. Acne of the face in adolescents was treated similarly. A significant number of children treated in this way have developed thyroid cancer 10–60 years later, and X-ray therapy for such benign conditions in childhood has long since been abandoned. Similarly the treatment by X-rays of an enlarged thymus gland or red birth-marks on the face or neck of infants may later give rise to cancer of the thyroid. In Japan survivors of the atomic bomb have, since the late 1950s, shown an increase in malignant thyroid nodules.

A pre-existing goitre, irrespective of its cause, does not seem to increase the risk of malignant change, and most thyroid cancers develop in a previously normal gland.

Points that may alert your doctor to the possibility of thyroid cancer are:

- a previous history of X-ray therapy to the head or neck;
- the sudden development of a lump, which may or may not be painful, in your thyroid gland;
- a lump in, or asymmetrical enlargement of, the thyroid particularly in a child or man (because thyroid disease is relatively uncommon in men);

- hoarseness of your voice;
- the finding of enlarged lymph glands in the neck in association with a goitre or a thyroid nodule;
- excessive hardness of the thyroid or the nodule.

Are there different types of thyroid cancer?

There are several different types of cancers that affect the thyroid gland and these can be separated into two main groups:

- those in which the cells are well differentiated and look like and behave in rather the same way as normal thyroid cells; and
- those in which the cells are not differentiated (anaplastic) and behave in a very unruly manner.

Differentiated cancers

In these the cells that have become malignant continue to look very much like normal thyroid cells and behave like them too. They continue to respond to the thyroid-stimulating hormone from the pituitary and they may continue to take up iodine (and radio-iodine) from the bloodstream. Therefore these tumours are relatively 'civilized'; they grow slowly and spread to distant parts of the body (metastasize) late. The fact that they often continue to take up radio-iodine makes the detection of secondary deposits (metastases) in other parts of the body easier and allows effective treatment to be given by irradiating the metastases with radio-iodine. Also if the secretion of TSH from the pituitary is reduced to negligible amounts by giving thyroxine by mouth, the stimulus for the cancer cells to grow is diminished.

Undifferentiated cancers

Less commonly the cells of a thyroid cancer are undifferentiated. These 'uncivilized' anaplastic cells, like anarchists, are uncontrolled and uncontrollable. They multiply rapidly and invade surrounding structures in the neck, which may make surgical removal difficult or impossible.

There are certain other forms of cancer that may involve the thyroid gland and these are mentioned for the sake of completeness.

Medullary cell cancer

A very rare form of cancer may develop from cells which, strictly speaking, are not thyroid cells at all but 'lodgers' living in the thyroid gland. These so-called medullary cells, also known as C cells or parafollicular cells, do not make or secrete thyroid hormones. They manufacture a hormone called calcitonin (hence 'C cells') which regulates the amount of calcium in your bones. They may also secrete other hormones that increase the activity of the intestines and cause diarrhoea. These rare medullary cell cancers tend to run in families and to be associated with small non-malignant tumours of the adrenal glands in the abdomen (phaeochromocytomas) that secrete excess adrenalin (epinephrine) and noradrenalin (norepinephrine)—hormones that cause high blood pressure. Because so rare, medullary cell cancers will not be considered further except to say that surgical removal of the malignant tumour in the neck and the associated benign phaeochromocytoma(s) in the abdomen is often successful.

Lymphomas

Sometimes the thyroid is the site of a malignant lymphoma, a tumour that arises from white corpuscles (lymphocytes or related cells) residing in the thyroid gland. Lymphomas are often fast growing so that the thyroid increases rapidly in size and may compress the windpipe to cause shortness of breath or a crowing noise (stridor) when you breathe out. These tumours are usually sensitive to X-ray treatment and chemotherapy.

Metastatic cancer

Sometimes the thyroid becomes the site of secondary deposits from a primary cancer in the lung, breast, or kidney but at this stage the underlying growth will usually have declared itself.

What happens to you in thyroid cancer?

If you develop the most common sort of thyroid cancer—the differentiated kind—the first thing you will probably notice is the development of a small lump in your thyroid. This lump is usually round and nodular, often hard to the touch, usually but not always painless, and may initially be no bigger than a pea. Your thyroid may previously have been perfectly normal or you may know that you have a goitre.

Sometimes more than one lump appears because these differentiated cancers may start in several different parts of the thyroid gland at the same time. The malignant cells may spread to a nearby lymph gland in your neck and this may be what takes you to your doctor to complain of a swollen gland in your neck, which is an enlarged painless lymph node and with little to suggest that the primary growth is in the thyroid gland itself.

Left untreated a differentiated thyroid cancer will eventually spread (metastasize) to other parts of your body, the malignant cells being carried in the bloodstream or the lymphatic system to your lungs, liver, or your bones. Not until there has been considerable destruction of a bone by a metastasis will you feel any bone pain. Sometimes the pain comes on suddenly if the involved bone breaks without any preceding fall or unusual force being applied (a 'pathological fracture'). Hoarseness of your voice may also occur if the malignant cells encroach on the nerves that activate your vocal cords.

The undifferentiated anaplastic type of thyroid cancer tends to occur in older people. The gland enlarges quite quickly and becomes generally tender. The highly malignant cells may invade the overlying skin, making it red as though it were inflamed. Deeper structures in your neck may be invaded so that on swallowing your thyroid gland does not move up and down in your neck as freely as it should. Huskiness of the voice is common.

How is cancer of the thyroid diagnosed?

The diagnosis is made on the basis of your doctor's clinical suspicion and confirmed mainly by a biopsy, either a needle biopsy and/or removal of the affected tissue at operation. Sometimes, in addition, a radioisotope scan may help to establish the diagnosis. Clinical suspicion will be aroused if there is:

- sudden enlargement of any part of an existing goitre;
- sudden development of a nodule or nodules in a previously normal thyroid gland or in a goitre;
- a history of previous X-ray therapy to the head, neck or chest;

- pain or discomfort in the thyroid gland in the absence of evidence of Hashimoto's or subacute viral thyroiditis (see Chapters 7 and 9);
- huskiness of the voice, although there are many more common causes of this.

A radio-iodine scan or a technetium scan, but preferably the former, may be helpful in deciding that cancer is probably *not* present but is less helpful in deciding that it is. Malignant tissue may fail to take up the isotope as avidly as do normal thyroid cells. Although many benign lumps do take up the isotope, unfortunately many do not and are also 'cold'. Thus if your lump takes up the isotope, it is unlikely to be a cancer. If your lump fails to do so, however, it could be either malignant or benign. A needle biopsy may settle the matter but if there is any doubt surgery will be recommended.

Tests of thyroid function will probably be done but these do not help in establishing the diagnosis and only very rarely is a thyroid cancer, even when it has spread widely, the cause of thyrotoxicosis.

An enlarged lymph node in the neck

There are many relatively trivial and also many serious causes for you developing an enlarged lymph node in the neck. Happily the less serious are much more common than the serious causes. They range from a simple sore throat or glandular fever (infective mononucleosis) to tuberculosis or cancer of various kinds. Examination by your doctor and simple investigations will usually establish the cause but sometimes more complicated tests are required including the removal of the lymph gland.

How is cancer of the thyroid treated?

Differentiated cancer

The treatment of a differentiated thyroid cancer is usually successful. At operation, while you are anaesthetized, the tissue under suspicion is removed and examined under the microscope. If this confirms cancer, your surgeon will probably remove all your thyroid gland (a total thyroidectomy). Thus not only is the malignant tissue removed but also the rest of the seemingly normal gland. This is done because of the possibility that other small areas of cancer may be present in other parts of the thyroid. In skilled hands a total thyroidectomy can usually be accomplished without damage to the nerves to your vocal cords and without loss of all the parathyroid glands (p. 43). The surgeon will remove any neighbouring lymph glands in your neck which may be the site of local spread. Some few weeks after you have recovered from the operation you will be given a therapeutic dose of radioactive iodine with the objective of killing off any residual thyroid cells—normal or malignant. This will mean being admitted to hospital where you will be nursed in a special room for about a week. After you have been given the radio-iodine, the radioactivity will be carefully monitored and you will be discharged from hospital when the radiation has fallen to the recommended level. You will be advised about when you can return to work and when you can resume non-essential contact with children and other adults.

Thereafter you will be given replacement therapy to make good your thyroid hormone deficiency. Either thyroxine (T_4) or triiodothyronine (T_3) may be prescribed for you. The dosage will be adjusted until the level of your thyroid-stimulating hormone is suppressed below normal, but not sufficient thyroid hormone will be given to make you hyperthyroid. By keeping the TSH level suppressed any remaining malignant thyroid cells are not exposed to its stimulating action and thus remain dormant.

After six or nine months your hospital doctor may wish to check that all is perfectly well with you. Nowadays your hospital doctor, at regular intervals of 6–12 months, may simply monitor your freedom from any recurrence of the cancer by measuring the level of thyroglobulin in your blood. This is a substance present in small amounts in the blood of normal people. In patients with a differentiated thyroid cancer, treated in the way described above, little or no thyroglobulin should be found in your blood because all the normal and malignant thyroid cells have been eradicated. Increased amounts will appear if there is a recurrence of your cancer. Thus your doctor may simply monitor your thyroglobulin level while you continue taking thyroxine to prevent thyroid deficiency and to suppress your TSH.

If the thyroglobulin level rises, your replacement thyroid hormone treatment is stopped for a few weeks until your TSH level has risen above the upper normal range. Then you are given a tracer dose of radio-iodine and a scan is done of your neck and your whole body. If any significant number of thyroid cells, normal or malignant, remain in the neck they will show up and so also will any significant number of differentiated cancerous cells that have formed secondary deposits elsewhere in your body.

If the scans show evidence of residual thyroid tissue, a further treatment dose of radio-iodine is given and the replacement treatment with thyroid hormone restarted.

Before measurement of the blood thyroglobulin level was introduced, radio-iodine scanning used to be, and in some centres still is, repeated annually so that any recurrence of the cancer could be detected early and treated with radio-iodine.

Undifferentiated thyroid cancer

In the early stages of an undifferentiated (anaplastic) thyroid cancer it may be possible to remove the growth surgically, but often the best treatment is deep X-ray therapy.

Here is an account by a woman patient who had a differentiated thyroid cancer. Initially this was not treated in an ideal way but happily all is well now.

When I was aged 35 a small painless lump appeared in my thyroid gland but I took no notice of it. Two years later I had my last (my third) child and during this pregnancy the lump increased in size. Not until I was 40 did the lump seem sufficiently large for me to draw my doctor's attention to it. At that time we were living abroad. The lump was removed surgically and I was told it was a cancer. I was given thyroxine tablets.

Four years later—we were still living in Africa—I noticed another lump in my thyroid gland on the other side. This time the surgeon removed all my thyroid gland and I was given more thyroid hormone to take by mouth.

When I was 46 we came back to England and I noticed a painless lump in the right side of my neck under the angle of my jaw. A radio-iodine scan showed it was thyroid issue—almost certainly malignant they said—in a lymph gland. I was operated on and several lymph glands containing cancer were removed. I was then given what my doctor said was a curative dose of radio-active iodine.

I'm now 56. Isotope scans were done each year until I was 50 but now my thyroglobulin is measured every 6 months. I have had no recurrence and certainly I feel fine taking 0.25 mg thyroxine daily.

Questions and Answers

*Q.*1 I have had many tests and have been told that the results are encouraging, but I have been advised to have an operation. I don't understand.

A. The tests may indicate that your thyroid is functioning normally, but the biopsy may still be equivocal and it may not be possible to be absolutely certain that this lump in your thyroid gland isn't malignant. The only way to be sure is to remove it. Even if it is a cancer, the outlook is very good.

*Q.*2 Will I have to go through all this again next year—I mean this radio-isotope scan to show I've not got any cancer left?

A. No, in future your absence of disease can be monitored by measuring a substance called thyroglobulin in a simple blood sample. Only if this test comes back positive will you have to have another radio-iodine scan.

*Q.*3 My dose of thyroxine has been increased. Does that mean I'm worse; that the cancer has come back?

A. Certainly not. Your dosage of thyroxine has been raised a little because the blood level of TSH, that stimulates any remaining thyroid cells, is not sufficiently suppressed.

*Q.*4 But won't increasing my thyroxine dose make me nervous and jumpy?

A. The aim is to increase the blood level of your thyroid hormone to the upper limit of normal, but not to a level that will upset you.

*Q.*5 Is it certain that I haven't got cancer?

A. Almost. The scan shows that you have a great many nodules in your thyroid, although you may only feel one, and that makes it much less likely to be malignant.

13

Thyroid problems in pregnancy and afterwards

Changes occur in your thyroid gland during pregnancy in parallel with the other major hormonal adjustments that occur during this time.

Pregnancy with a normal thyroid gland

During pregnancy in any woman with a normal thyroid there is a tendency for the gland to enlarge. This is why in ancient Egypt a fine thread used to be tied round the neck of a young bride; when the thread broke it was evidence that she had become pregnant. The increase in size, if it occurs at all, is usually slight. Why the thyroid becomes larger is not known for certain but it may be related to a relative degree of iodine deficiency which develops because the baby will take iodine from its mother, and during pregnancy the mother loses more iodine in her urine than normally. Another factor may be that certain hormones formed in the afterbirth (the placenta) may mildly stimulate your thyroid gland.

Any slight enlargement of your thyroid during pregnancy is likely to be of no consequence but you should ensure that you have an adequate—neither too little nor too much—intake of iodine by using sea salt or iodized salt in cooking and at the table, and eat sea fish at least once weekly.

Some of the thyroid function tests change during pregnancy. The levels of total T_4 and total T_3 tend to rise because there is an increase in the level of the hormone-binding globulin (p. 125) as a result of the increase in the female hormone (oestrogen) during pregnancy. However the unbound free T_4 and free T_3, which are the biologically active hormones, do not increase; indeed during the last 3 months of pregnancy they may actually fall. These laboratory changes are not important to you if your thyroid is normal, but they are if you suffered from an overactivity or an underactivity of your thyroid gland before you became pregnant or if either was first diagnosed during your pregnancy.

Pregnancy and the overactive thyroid

If you have untreated hyperthyroidism, you are unlikely to become pregnant. However once your overactive thyroid is controlled by an antithyroid drug or you are cured (made euthyroid again) by either surgery or radio-iodine, your fertility will be restored to normal. If you become pregnant while you are taking an antithyroid drug (see p. 38), this treatment will be continued in the smallest effective dose during the pregnancy and stopped, except in very florid cases, during the last 4-6 weeks before your expected date of delivery. In most cases it is possible to stop the treatment towards the end of your pregnancy because the auto-immune disorder that causes your Graves' disease tends to lessen during this time and the thyrotoxicosis becomes milder. Alternatively surgical removal of seven-eighths of your thyroid can be done during the middle 3 months of your pregnancy, when it is safe to operate on you without harming your baby or the risk of inducing a miscarriage.

Sometimes thyroid overactivity, nearly always due to Graves' disease, develops *during* pregnancy. The diagnosis is not always easy because some of the symptoms of thyroid overactivity—such as an increased heart rate and palpitations, feeling hot, increased perspiration, nervousness, and tiredness—may also occur in pregnant women with a normal thyroid gland. Some hyperthyroid pregnant women fail to gain weight to the degree expected.

How is thyrotoxicosis diagnosed during pregnancy?

Because of the changes that occur in thyroid function tests during pregnancy, the diagnosis must rest on the level of the *free* thyroid hormones and a low TSH level. A radio-iodine uptake test (p. 19) must not be done during pregnancy because the isotope would also be taken up by your baby's thyroid gland.

How will I be treated?

If you develop Graves' disease during pregnancy you will be treated with an antithyroid drug, with or without subtotal thyroidectomy in the middle 3 months of the pregnancy, as described in Chapter 4. If you are not operated on, it will probably be possible, as explained above, to stop your antithyroid medication during the last 6 weeks of your pregnancy.

What will happen after I have had my baby?

If you have not been operated on, your antithyroid drug will have to be restarted but it will be secreted in your milk. Thus it is usually advised that you should not breast-feed your baby. However, the amounts of carbimazole or methimazole present in your milk are usually small and there is no absolute reason why you should not breast-feed provided a careful eye is kept on your baby who may need some blood tests from time to time.

Pregnancy and the underactive thyroid

Infertility is also common in women who have an underactive thyroid gland. Once the thyroid deficiency is corrected, however, normal fertility is restored. It is most important, if you have an underactive thyroid gland and are being treated with thyroid hormone replacement therapy, that you continue this during your pregnancy and afterwards. Just because your total T_4 and T_3 increase above the normal non-pregnant range this is no reason to reduce or stop your dose of hormone replacement. Furthermore, in some hypothyroid people on treatment, the thyroid-stimulating hormone (TSH) rises during pregnancy and this is an indication to slightly *increase* the dosage of your replacement therapy.

Thyroid problems after delivery

Abnormalities of thyroid function are quite common after delivery, and usually occur about 3 months after your baby is born. During this postpartum period either mild hyperthyroidism, hypothyroidism, or thyroid overactivity followed by underactivity may occur. Recent studies indicate that as many as about 15 per cent of women, particularly those who have certain thyroid antibodies (microsomal antibodies, see p. 121) present in their blood when they become pregnant, develop some disorder of thyroid function during the first 3–6 months after having a baby. Short-lived thyroid overactivity alone, or transient thyroid overactivity followed by short-lived underactivity are less common than hypothyroidism alone.

The symptoms produced by these abnormalities are seldom recognized because many women accept them as the consequences of having to look after a new baby and having to run their home. Often the thyroid over- or underactivity is so short lived that no treatment is necessary.

What happens if I become hypothyroid after delivery?

In some women the symptoms of underactivity of the thyroid gland, characterized by fatigue, weakness, depression, failure to lose weight, impairment of memory, and lack of ability to concentrate, are incorrectly attributed by them, or ascribed by their doctor, to postpartum 'blues'. Treatment with thyroxine can prove beneficial. In some women the thyroxine replacement is only required temporarily, but in about a quarter it is required on a permanent basis.

What happens if I develop hyperthyroidism after delivery?

Usually this is so short-lived that no treatment is required but a beta-blocker (p. 35) will help relieve any symptoms. Postpartum hyper-thyroidism is also known as 'silent thyroiditis'—'silent' not because there are no symptoms, but because the thyroid gland is not painful or tender and seldom is it obviously enlarged. The cause of this thyroid overactivity is almost certainly due to a type of auto-immune thyroiditis quite different from Graves' disease. Radio-iodine scanning shows reduced uptake of the isotope, but this test can only be done if you stop breast-feeding for 4 days because the radioactive iodine may be secreted in your milk. Silent thyroiditis is discussed further in Chapter 14 (p. 107).

Will my baby be all right?

In most instances when you have medical treatment for an overactive or underactive thyroid gland during your pregnancy, your baby will be perfectly all right and if anything does go wrong it can always be put right because your doctor will be on the look-out for it.

Neonatal hyperthyroidism

Thyroid overactivity (congenital hyperthyroidism) in a new-born baby is very rare. It occurs only when the baby's mother had Graves' disease during the pregnancy or was in the past treated for Graves' disease. The cause of your baby's hyperthyroidism is the thyroid-stimulating anti-bodies that you have in your blood and which passed, during your pregnancy, to your baby. These stimulating antibodies may persist in your blood even though your Graves' disease was treated and cured long ago.

In fact very few babies (less than 1 in 100) of previously thyrotoxic mothers are affected but are somewhat more likely to be so if you had severe eye complications (Chapter 5) or pretibial myxoedema (p. 31)—both findings which are sometimes associated with high levels of thyroid-stimulating antibodies that may persist in your blood.

If you were treated with an antithyroid drug during pregnancy it is unlikely your baby will be born hyperthyroid because the carbimazole or methimazole will cross the placenta and suppress your baby's thyroid gland.

Can they tell if my baby will be born with hyperthyroidism?

In any woman with a past or present history of Graves' disease, a careful watch will be kept on your baby before it is born. Congenital hyper-thyroidism may be suspected if *in utero* your baby's heart rate is unduly fast or if your baby grows abnormally fast as measured by an ultrasound scan. Your doctor may be alerted to the possibility of your baby being thyrotoxic by finding a high level of thyroid-stimulating antibodies in your blood. When this test is available it should be done if you have Graves' disease in pregnancy or had it in the past. If there is evidence of intra-uterine thyrotoxicosis, the overactive thyroid of your baby can be treated by giving you an antithyroid drug. During this treatment you can be prevented from becoming hypothyroid by giving you thyroxine which barely crosses the placenta and thus will not affect your baby.

What if my baby has congenital hyperthyroidism?

If, as rarely happens, your baby has congenital hyperthyroidism it will have an unduly fast heart rate and be restless. Minimal eye signs may be present but the other main features are failure to thrive and gain weight despite an enormous appetite, flushing of the skin and possibly diarrhoea. Your baby's thyroid gland is likely to be enlarged but this is not easy to detect at this age. The diagnosis can quickly be confirmed by measuring your baby's thyroid hormone level but it must be remembered that a somewhat raised T_4 level is normal at birth.

Treatment is given with small doses of iodine and an antithyroid drug. Fortunately neonatal thyrotoxicosis is self-limiting because the thyroid-stimulating antibodies from you persist in your baby for only a few weeks or months. Thus active treatment is required only during this time.

Could my baby be born thyroid deficient?

This too is very rare. If you were given too much of an antithyroid drug during your pregnancy to control your Graves' disease, in theory your baby could be born with a suppressed thyroid gland.

If you developed hypothyroidism during your pregnancy and were treated for this, you need not worry. Do not forget that your baby has its own thyroid gland that started working when it was an 8-week-old fetus.

However, like every other baby, yours must be tested to exclude thyroid deficiency between the fifth and tenth day after birth (p. 69) because the more common causes of hypothyroidism could affect your baby like anyone else's.

Questions and Answers

Q.1 After my first baby was born, I had thyroid deficiency for about 6 months. Is this likely to happen again if I have another child?

A. Yes, unfortunately it is, particularly as you have thyroid antibodies in your blood.

Q.2 Would it be better to have an operation for my Graves' disease even though I'm pregnant or go on taking carbimazole all the way through?

A. Thyrotoxicosis in pregnant women can usually be easily controlled with a small dose of an anti-thyroid drug such as carbimazole or methimazole, which can be stopped a few weeks before delivery. You are likely to need to restart it a few weeks later. Surgery nowadays is usually only recommended during pregnancy if it is very difficult to control the Graves' disease or if you would need a large dose of the antithyroid drug to do so.

Q.3 Might there be problems in feeding the baby?

A. Only because the carbimazole might appear in your milk, but the concentration is so small that it is unlikely to harm the baby.

*Q.*4   Is there any guarantee that the carbimazole will cure my hyperthyroidism?

A.   Unfortunately not, but it is usually very effective.

*Q.*5   My obstetrician has told me that my thyroxine level is too high and he
wondered whether I should reduce my dose of thyroxine.

A.   The level of *total* thyroxine in your blood is high due to the pregnancy,
but that is to be expected and does not necessarily mean that you need to
reduce the dose. Measurements of the *free* thyroxine and TSH are usually
normal in this situation. Only if the free thyroxine is too high and the
TSH suppressed would your dose of thyroxine need to be reduced.

14

Miscellaneous disorders of the thyroid gland

A number of miscellaneous disorders of the thyroid gland, not dealt with elsewhere in this book or in need of further consideration are discussed in this chapter.

Pituitary diseases and the thyroid

Although the relationship of the pituitary gland, its secretion of thyroid-stimulating hormone (TSH), and the thyroid gland have been discussed in Chapter 1, little mention has been made of the thyroid disorders that may develop as a consequence of pituitary disease.

Excessive secretion of TSH

Overactivity of the pituitary gland with increased secretion of TSH is a rare cause of thyroid overactivity (p. 55). The clue that leads to your doctor diagnosing this is that you are thyrotoxic with a raised level of thyroid hormones in your blood but surprisingly the TSH level is normal or raised—not suppressed as is usually the case due to operation of the feedback mechanism (p. 5).

Although antithyroid drugs will reduce the excessive production of thyroid hormones and render you euthyroid, this treatment will not cure the condition. Attention has to be given to why your pituitary gland is secreting too much TSH and correcting this.

Reduced secretion of TSH

Failure of the pituitary gland to secrete enough TSH is more common and is the cause of secondary thyroid failure. Lack of enough TSH reduces the secretion of thyroid hormones from your thyroid gland, and causes a clinical picture very similar to that which follows primary failure of the thyroid gland (Chapter 8). This picture is often modified, however, by additional features resulting from the diminished secretion of other pituitary hormones that influence growth, sexual development and function, and the adrenal glands.

Reduced secretion of TSH is usually due to either a tumour or some other damage to your pituitary gland. Therefore in addition to failure of your thyroid, there is failure of other endocrine glands. If a tumour of the pituitary is the cause, it may induce local symptoms in your head, such as headaches and/or visual disturbances.

If a tumour is present, treatment must be directed at this and replacement therapy given, not only to make good the thyroid deficiency but the deficiencies of the other endocrine glands that are controlled by the pituitary such as the ovaries in women, the testes in men, and the adrenal glands—all of which may have become underactive too.

Here is an account of the illness of a woman who suffered destruction of her pituitary gland as a result of an unhappy obstetric event. In pregnancy the pituitary gland enlarges and is very dependent on a good blood supply. As we shall learn this patient's blood supply to her pituitary was jeopardized when she had her baby.

I'm now 39 years old. I got married at the age of 26 after training to be a nurse. My husband is a lawyer and we moved to the Middle East where I had Benjamin when I was 28. Immediately after he was born I had an enormous haemorrhage. The head-nurse told me that my haemoglobin fell to 7g/100 ml whereas my normal level is 14 g/100 ml. There were no facilities to give me a blood transfusion which I'm sure they would have done at home. I couldn't feed Benjie because I had no milk.

My periods never came back properly; I just had the odd one, very light, every now and then. Although we take no precautions, I've never become pregnant again. I put on a certain amount of weight and I lost my libido; I just wasn't interested in sex any more. I began to feel tired all the time and lost my sparkle. I also became constipated which I'd never been before, and when we returned to England when Benjie was 4 I couldn't stand the cold.

I went to my doctor in England and she pointed out that the hair under my arms had disappeared and my pubic hair was very sparse; something I hadn't noticed because it happened so slowly. She quickly confirmed that I was hypothyroid but was surprised that my TSH level was not raised at all. I think it was that which made her realize my pituitary had packed up. She sent me to a specialist who did a lot of tests one morning. He found that my ovaries and my adrenal glands, as well as my thyroid, were not working properly because most of my pituitary had been knocked off when I had that ghastly postpartum haemorrhage. As a result my pituitary no longer produces enough TSH or the hormones that should activate my ovaries and adrenals.

I'm feeling fine now—better than I have for ages. Of course I have to take a lot of pills but I'm used to that and never forget. I take thyroxine for my thyroid, a steroid called hydrocortisone twice a day for my adrenals, and oestrogens—hormone replacement therapy really—for my inactive ovaries.

Silent thyroiditis

This is a rare cause of hyperthyroidism. It is called 'silent' because the thyroid gland is not tender as in subacute viral thyroiditis (Chapter 9) nor is it much enlarged. The exact cause is not known; it may in some cases be due to a virus infection but in most it is a short-lived auto-immune disorder. It occurs more often in women than men, and is particularly common in the postpartum period (see p. 101). It has been found more commonly in North America, where it is the cause of hyperthyroidism in 10 per cent of patients, than in Europe.

What happens in silent thyroiditis?

If you develop silent thyroiditis you will become thyrotoxic (p. 29) but the degree of this is seldom severe, nor will you have eye complications. The level of thyroid hormones in your blood will be raised and your TSH depressed. However the most important finding is that a technetium or radio-iodine scan will show a *reduced* uptake of the isotope by your thyroid gland. This cardinal difference distinguishes silent thyroiditis from Graves' disease.

How will I be treated?

Silent thyroiditis is a relatively short-lived condition that remits spontaneously. If your thyrotoxicosis is mild, no treatment or a beta-blocker is all that is required. In more severe cases a short course of an antithyroid drug is used. The more rigorous treatments used for the treatment of Graves' disease (Chapter 4), such as radio-iodine or thyroidectomy, are quite inappropriate for you because in due course you will get better.

Are there any after effects?

Sometimes silent thyroiditis is followed by hypothyroidism and this is most often seen in postpartum women (p. 100). The phase of thyroid deficiency is usually short-lived but in about a quarter of patients it is permanent and this will mean life-long thyroxine replacement treatment.

Thyroid crisis or storm

This is a rare condition in which a patient with thyrotoxicosis has a sudden and severe exacerbation of their hyperthyroid symptoms. This usually comes about as a result of some intercurrent illness such as influenza, a sore throat, or pneumonia in a person who does not know they are thyrotoxic or in a patient whose hyperthyroidism is not being adequately controlled. In the old days a thyroid crisis or storm was not uncommon when surgeons operated on patients who had not been properly prepared by modern methods for the operation and had not been rendered euthyroid. An excess of thyroid hormones was released into the bloodstream as the surgeon handled the incompletely prepared thyroid gland during its subtotal removal.

What happens in a thyroid crisis?

The excess of thyroid hormones in the blood induces a fever, a very rapid irregular heart beat (atrial fibrillation), heart failure, profound sweating with loss of body water, a state of shock with a low blood pressure, and mental confusion or delirium. The outcome may be fatal.

How is a thyroid crisis treated?

The best 'treatment' is prevention, but this is not always possible if the patient does not know she is thyrotoxic. If a thyroid storm does occur, treatment with potassium iodide by mouth, antithyroid drugs, and beta-blockers as well as intravenous replacement of fluid must be prompt.

Apathetic hyperthyroidism

This is a very rare, and rather mysterious, condition that occurs only in older patients, usually in neglected, undiagnosed and therefore untreated hyperthyroidism of some duration. The clinical picture is such that apathetic thyrotoxicosis may easily escape recognition because it is so divergent from the ordinary hyperthyroidism seen in younger patients.

The patient is emotionally flat and depressed in contrast to the usual picture of anxiety and emotional over-alertness. Instead of being restless the patient with apathetic thyrotoxicosis is lethargic and underactive, and often has a poor appetite. Although there may be a history or evidence of weight loss, the patient appears bloated. Seldom is there marked thyroid enlargement or any eye complications. The pulse may be slow or normal as opposed to the expected increase in rate. Sometimes the illness is attributed to the patient getting old, to some hidden cancer, or to depression.

Apathetic hyperthyroidism responds well to antithyroid drugs but as these may not induce a permanent cure radio-iodine is usually given once the thyroid overactivity has been controlled.

The 'sick euthyroid' syndrome

This is not a true 'illness' that you need be concerned about; it is more a problem and matter of interest to your doctor. If you become really ill from any cause whatsoever the level of total and free T_3 in your blood may drop below normal and in severe cases so may your total and free T_4. This may suggest to your doctor that you are thyroid deficient, but you are not because the level of TSH in your blood is not raised. As you recover from whatever non-thyroid illness you have, the level of the thyroid hormones returns to normal.

Riedel's thyroiditis

This is an extremely rare condition in which the thyroid gland becomes replaced by scarring fibrous tissue. The thyroid may be tender and feels as hard as wood. The condition is also known as ligneous (woody) or invasive fibrous thyroiditis.

The gland becomes attached to the overlying skin and to deeper structures in the neck so that your windpipe may be constricted and involvement of the nerves to your vocal cords makes your voice weak or husky. Swallowing may be difficult. Without a biopsy it may be difficult for your doctor to distinguish this condition from an undifferentiated anaplastic cancer (p. 91), and an operation is usually required to relieve the constriction of the windpipe.

Riedel's thyroiditis may be associated with a similar fibrosis affecting the covering of the intestines (peritoneal fibrosis), structures in the back of your abdomen (retroperitoneal fibrosis), the duct that carries bile from the liver to the intestines (sclerosing cholangitis), or structures in the centre of the chest (mediastinal fibrosis). The cause of this very uncommon condition is unknown.

Suppurative thyroiditis

This too is very uncommon. In suppurative thyroiditis your thyroid gland becomes infected with pus-forming bacteria such as staphylococci which are the cause of boils. The thyroid gland becomes acutely inflamed and very painful. You will have a high fever and be very ill, often with the infection spreading to other parts of your body. The response to an appropriate antibiotic is usually rapid.

Questions and Answers

Q.1   When my grandmother had her thyroid removed for Graves' disease when she was quite young, she tells me she had to wait until the winter before they'd operate. Why was that, and how is it I am told that I can have my operation later this summer?

A.   In those days it wasn't easy to be certain that a patient's thyrotoxicosis was controlled before surgery was done. Your grandmother would have been admitted to hospital and given Lugol's iodine for about 10 days. Her pulse, particularly when she was asleep at night, would have been recorded, and she would be expected to have gained weight before it was safe to operate. It was also found safer to operate in cold weather than in hot. Nowadays you can be prepared for the operation much more safely and it will not be performed until your thyroid overactivity has been properly controlled.

Q.2   My pituitary gland was damaged when I had a postpartum haemorrhage. Will it ever recover?

A.   Sometimes it does if the damage is slight, but if the haemorrhage was severe, there is little chance of recovery.

*Q.*3   First I was told that I had Sheehan's syndrome, and now that I have hypopituitarism. Are these the same thing?

A.   Yes. The late Professor Sheehan of Liverpool first described the association between haemorrhage following childbirth and the later development
of failure of the pituitary gland.

*Q.*4   Have I got to take all these tablets for the rest of my life? It'll cost a
fortune.

A.   It is essential that you take the hydrocortisone and thyroxine for the rest of
your life, although the female hormone tablets may be stopped when you
are 65 or so. They won't cost you anything with the British National
Health Service because medicines for endocrine deficiency are dispensed
free of charge to the patient. In other health care systems you may have to
pay for the tablets, but they are not very expensive and they are essential
for your continued well-being.

15

Other diseases associated with thyroid disorders

Certain people and certain families appear to be more prone to auto-immune diseases than others. The reason for this is not yet fully understood, but patients with auto-immune thyroid disease are more likely to develop other auto-immune disorders. For example if you develop Hashimoto's thyroiditis you may find that your grandmother had Graves' hyperthyroidism. In other words two different types of auto-immune thyroid disease are occurring in the same family but skipping a generation as often happens. Auto-immune thyroid diseases certainly run in families but so also do other auto-immune disorders although not all members of a family are so affected. There are several other auto-immune diseases that you should know about because a relative of yours may have got one or you, already with an auto-immune thyroid disease, could possibly one day develop a non-thyroid auto-immune disorder, uncommon though this may be.

The following are auto-immune disorders that may sometimes be associated with auto-immune thyroid disease.

Pernicious (Addisonian) anaemia

This is a particular type of anaemia which should no longer be called 'pernicious' because it is so easily treated. In Addisonian anaemia (named after the physician at Guy's Hospital who first described it in 1855), the body makes antibodies against certain cells in the wall of the stomach. These cells secrete a substance which promotes the absorption of Vitamin B_{12} from the intestinal tract and Vitamin B_{12} is essential for the making of red blood corpuscles. Addisonian anaemia is easily corrected by giving injections of Vitamin B_{12} every 6 weeks or so.

Diabetes mellitus

Sugar diabetes, particularly the type that starts in young people and requires insulin for its control, occurs with an increased incidence in the families of patients who have auto-immune thyroid diseases. Diabetes mellitus is probably, at least in part, an auto-immune disease caused by antibodies attacking the cells in the pancreas that secrete the hormone insulin. The presenting symptoms of juvenile or ir_ulin-dependent diabetes, which may come on quite suddenly, are the passing of large volumes of urine, increased thirst, tiredness, and weight loss. Treatment is by diet and injections of insulin.

Addison's disease of the adrenal glands

Lying just above the kidneys are two small endocrine glands—the adrenal or suprarenal glands—which secrete steroid hormones like cortisone. These hormones are essential to life and regulate the blood pressure and the response to infections, stress, physical accidents, and surgery. Failure of the adrenal glands was described in 1855 by the same physician, Dr Addison, who described pernicious anaemia. The adrenal glands may be destroyed by tuberculosis but nowadays the most common cause is auto-immune destruction of the adrenal cells. Addison's adrenal failure is characterized by extreme weakness and fatigue, a low blood pressure, and darkening of the skin. It responds well to replacement therapy with cortisone and related steroids taken by mouth.

Polymyalgia rheumatica and giant-cell arteritis

These two diseases are related. The first is characterized by nasty pain in the muscles and joints. Giant-cell arteritis, or cranial arteritis as it is also called, gives rise to headaches, fever, and general malaise. Either or both of these conditions may occasionally be associated with hypothyroidism caused by Hashimoto's disease and may occur before or after the hypothyroidism declares itself.

Dyslexia

It appears that dyslexia is more common in families with auto-immune thyroid disease than in the population at large. Children with dyslexia may show a delay in their ability to read and later have difficulty with spelling and writing. These children are by no means stupid and often are very bright but because of their handicap they fall behind at school. Boys are more often affected than girls and tend to be left-handed.

Vitiligo

This is a skin disorder, also known as leucoderma (white skin), in which patches of white skin devoid of normal pigment develop. Vitiligo is a common associate of all auto-immune diseases and may be looked upon as a 'marker' or an indicator of some auto-immune disorder that may not develop for several years.

Myasthenia gravis

This is a rare muscle disorder caused by an auto-immune disturbance. It occurs about ten times more commonly in patients with Graves' disease than in the general population. Often it first affects the muscles of the eyes which leads to double vision. Later other muscles in the limbs or trunk may become involved. As the day progresses the patient experiences increasing weakness, and the more you try to do the weaker and more tired you become. There may be difficulty in swallowing, the voice becomes nasal, and breathing may become a struggle. The response to treatment is usually satisfactory.

Let one of our patients tell her story. She started with Graves' disease; then developed diabetes, only later to have Addisonian anaemia associated with vitiligo and ended up with hypothyroidism due to Hashimoto's disease.

I'm now aged 55. I trained as a lawyer but all my working life I've been in local government, in the tax department of one of the London boroughs. At the age of 12 I developed Graves' disease. I remember eating like a horse, but despite this I lost a lot of weight. My eyes became slightly starey. I was very clumsy and was always dropping things. My overactive thyroid was brought under control with antithyroid tablets, and everything was all right until at the age of 17 I began to lose weight again. I was very thirsty and used to take a jug of water to bed with me. My sleep was disturbed by having to get up several times at night to pass urine. Our doctor found that I'd developed diabetes, and this was treated with diet and twice daily insulin injections which I soon got used to. When I was 30 I was made deputy head of my department. Normally I'm pretty lively, but I became tired and my aunt commented on how pale I'd become. I'd also developed some funny white patches on my forearms. The doctor at the hospital where I go for my diabetes found I'd developed Addisonian anaemia. This quickly responded to injections of Vitamin B_{12} which I was given by our family doctor but I could have given them to myself as I'm used to injecting myself with insulin. I remained very well until I was aged about 45 when I began to feel the cold terribly and used to complain to the engineer at the Town Hall where I worked about the temperature in my office. He took no notice of me and I wore thicker clothes in a vain attempt to keep warm. Not until the next winter did I mention this to my family doctor and he spotted that I'd become thyroid deficient. Apparently I'd developed another sort of thyroid trouble called Hashimoto's disease but there was no swelling in my neck like there was when I had Graves' disease. The Hashimoto's was put right by giving me thyroxine. I feel fine now. I take my thyroid tablets every day, have my vitamin injection every month and give myself insulin injections twice daily.

Now you will understand why your doctor may do tests unrelated to your thyroid condition to be sure you have not got some other incipient auto-immune disorder, such as Addisonian anaemia, which may declare itself later on in your life.

Questions and Answers

Q.1   My grandmother says she had myxoedema 20 years ago; she's on
       thyroxine. Now I've got an overactive thyroid gland. Is there any
       connection?

A.   Yes, there probably is. Your grandmother and you both have auto-
       immune thyroid diseases of different kinds, and this does tend to run in
       families.

Q.2   I'm 50 years old and I've had Hashimoto's thyroiditis for years. I've been
       told that now I've got Addisonian anaemia. What is going to happen to
       me next?

A.   The chances of you developing some other auto-immune disease are very
       remote.

Glossary of terms

Addison's disease: this disease is the consequence of failure of the adrenal glands, usually caused by an auto-immune disorder. It may be associated with Hashimoto's thyroiditis.

Addisonian anaemia: a type of anaemia, also known as pernicious anaemia before effective treatment became available, caused by an auto-immune disorder which prevents absorption of Vitamin B_{12} from the intestine and may be associated with Hashimoto's thyroiditis (see Vitamin B_{12} below).

Adrenal glands: two small endocrine glands which lie on top of your kidneys and secrete cortisone-like steroid hormones. Normal function is essential to life.

Agranulocytosis: a disappearance of granulocytes (neutrophil white corpuscles) from the peripheral blood. This opens the door to infections. Agranulocytosis may rarely occur as a side-effect of treatment with antithyroid and several other types of drugs.

Anaplastic: a word used to describe very undifferentiated cancer cells which are aggressively malignant.

Antibodies: chemicals (proteins) that are formed in the body in response to invasion by any foreign protein (antigen). Auto-antibodies which react with 'self' are important in the causation of Graves' disease and Hashimoto's thyroiditis, and many other auto-immune disorders.

Antithyroid drugs: these drugs, such as carbimazole, methimazole, and propylthiouracil, suppress hormone manufacture by the cells of the thyroid gland.

Apathetic hyperthyroidism: an uncommon form of hyperthyroidism usually seen only in old people.

Auto-immune disease: a disease that results from the body making antibodies which attack normal cells or tissues in your body.

Benign: not malignant or cancerous.

Beta-adrenergic blocking drugs: these slow the heart rate, reduce palpitations and sweating, and improve some other features of thyroid activity but do not cure the underlying disease.

Beta-blockers: a colloquial name for beta-adrenergic blocking drugs.

Biopsy: a term used to describe removal of a small piece of tissue in order to examine it under the microscope. A biopsy may be made with a fine needle or at a surgical operation (an open biopsy).

Calcitonin: a hormone secreted by the medullary, C- or parafollicular cells that reside in the thyroid gland but are not of thyroid origin, and which influences the calcium level in your bones.

Carbimazole: an antithyroid drug.

Carcinoma: cancer. A differentiated carcinoma of the thyroid gland is one of the malignant diseases most amenable to treatment. An undifferentiated (anaplastic) carcinoma is more invasive.

Carrier-proteins: substances to which the thyroid hormones are loosely attached as they are transported round the body in the bloodstream (see thyroxine-binding globulin).

CAT scan: computer assisted tomography is a special type of X-ray examination, used in thyroid disorders to examine particularly the eye changes in Graves' disease and sometimes a retrosternal goitre, and compression or displacement of the windpipe.

Cholesterol: a particular type of fat found in the bloodstream. The level may be raised in hypothyroidism and decreased in hyperthyroidism, but is also affected by many other factors.

Chronic lymphocytic goitre: another name for Hashimoto's thyroiditis.

'Cold' nodule: a nodule in the thyroid gland that does not take up a radioisotope such as technetium or radio-iodine.

Congenital: existing at birth. A baby may be born with congenital hypothyroidism.

Corticosteroids: also called 'steroids', are cortisone-like hormones secreted by the adrenal (suprarenal) glands and as drugs are used to suppress an auto-immune response.

Cortisone: a corticosteroid drug now largely replaced by prednisone, prednisolone, or methylprednisolone.

Cretinism: thyroid deficiency occurring in an infant or child and associated with impaired mental development.

CT scan: see CAT scan.

Cyst: a hollow tumour, usually benign, which may contain fluid.

Decompression: surgical decompression of the bony orbits, in which the eyes lie, may be necessary to reduce the intra-orbital pressure in severe ophthalmopathy.

De Quervain's thyroiditis: the same as subacute viral thyroiditis.

Diffuse toxic goitre: another name for Graves' or von Basedow's disease.

Diplopia: double vision.

Dyshormonogenesis: a defect in one or more of the several chemical steps that take place in the manufacture of thyroid hormones. The defect varies in severity and may be a rare cause of thyroid underactivity and/or a goitre in infancy or childhood.

Dyslexia: a disorder of reading and writing that occurs in children.

Endemic goitre: when more than 20 per cent of a population being surveyed have a goitre, the goitre is said to be endemic.

Endocrine gland: a gland that forms and secretes hormones into the bloodstream. These chemical messengers affect cells and tissues far removed from where they are produced.

Euthyroid: this means that you have a normal level of thyroid hormones in your blood. You do not have over- or underactivity of your thyroid gland.

Exophthalmos: also known as proptosis. This means a protrusion of the eyeballs which are pushed forwards. A feature of Graves' ophthalmopathy.

Exophthalmometer: an instrument for measuring the degree of protrusion of your eyeballs.

Fibrosis: the deposition of fibrous connective tissue (scarring) in an organ that has been subjected to injury, usually inflammation, as may occur in the thyroid gland late in the course of Hashimoto's thyroiditis.

Free thyroxine level: this test measures the tiny amount of thyroxine that is present in the water of the blood, and which is a fraction of the very much larger amount that is loosely bound to the thyroxine-binding carrier-proteins. The advantage of measuring the *unbound 'free'* thyroxine is that the level is less influenced by changes in the amount of the carrier-proteins. The normal reference range for the free T_4 will depend on the exact technique used but, in round figures, is usually about 9–25 picomolecules per litre (pmol/L). Levels greater than 26 pmol/L occur in most cases of hyperthyroidism, and below 8 pmol/L in thyroid deficiency. The more severe the thyrotoxicosis the higher will be the free T_4 level and the more severe the hypothyroidism the lower the free T_4.

Occasionally the free T_4 test gives misleading results if certain interfering antibodies or an unusual albumin carrier-protein are present in your blood. Low levels may sometimes occur in a variety of non-thyroidal illnesses (see 'sick euthyroid' syndrome).

Free thyroxine index: this is not really a test in its own right. It is a mathematical calculation derived from the total thyroxine level and the T_3-resin-binding test. It makes allowance for alterations, upwards or downwards, in the proteins that carry your thyroxine and indirectly reflects the amount of thyroxine which is unattached to protein and floating free in the water of the blood. It is this free thyroxine that determines your thyroid status. It is for this reason that in many centres measurement of the free thyroxine is now used as a first-line test of thyroid function.

Free triiodothyronine level: this test measures the level of unbound 'free' T_3 in your blood. In normal people the reference range is of the order of about 3–9 pmol/L but varies slightly according to the technique used. The free T_3 is particularly useful in the diagnosis of hyperthyroidism because it may rise, some weeks or months, before the free thyroxine (fT_4) level does. Indeed there are some patients with thyrotoxicosis who never develop a raised thyroxine level (so-called T_3-toxicosis). The free T_3 is less useful than the free T_4 in diagnosing hypothyroidism, because the failing thyroid gland finds it easier to produce triiodothyronine and the level of T_3 falls later than the T_4 level. Low free T_3 levels are common in patients suffering from any non-thyroidal physical or psychiatric disease (see 'euthyroid sick' syndrome).

Goitre: any enlargement of the thyroid gland is called a goitre. The word is spelt goiter in the United States.

Graves' disease: an auto-immune disorder of the thyroid gland, named after the Irish physician who described it, that causes overactivity and increased levels of T_4 and/or T_3 in the blood (see also Von Basedow's disease).

Hashimoto's thyroiditis: an auto-immune disorder of the thyroid gland, named after the Japanese pathologist who first described it, which may cause thyroid enlargement (a goitre) and later underactivity of the gland (hypothyroidism).

Hashitoxicosis: a temporary episode of hyperthyroidism in a patient with Hashimoto's thyroiditis.

Hormone: a chemical substance made in an endocrine gland that is secreted into the bloodstream and affects tissues elsewhere in the body.

Hormone replacement therapy (HRT): this is the use of a hormone given to treat a condition in which the natural hormone is deficient. HRT, however, is usually used to describe the administration of ovarian hormones (oestrogens) for women at the time of the menopause.

'Hot' nodule: a nodule in the thyroid gland that actively takes up a tracer dose of a radioisotope to a greater degree than the surrounding thyroid tissue does.

Hyperthyroidism: overactivity of the thyroid gland which is characterized by certain symptoms and signs, a raised level of T_4 and/or T_3 and a suppressed TSH level in the blood.

Hypopituitarism: underactivity of the pituitary gland. This may affect just one, many or all the different hormones secreted by the gland, including the thyroid-stimulating hormone (TSH).

Hypothalamus: the hypothalamus is a small endocrine gland located in the brain close to the pituitary and secretes a number of different hormones. One of these is the thyrotrophin-releasing hormone (TRH) which stimulates the TSH-secreting cells in the pituitary.

Hypothyroidism: a condition in which the thyroid gland fails to secrete enough hormones.

Iodine: this element is an essential constituent of the thyroid hormones and is obtained from your diet. It is found in sea-fish, milk and other dairy products, and some vegetables.

Isotope: the form of an element with a slightly different atomic weight but the same chemical properties. Radioactive isotopes of iodine and technetium are used in the diagnosis of thyroid disorders and radio-iodine is also used in the treatment.

Isthmus: this is the little bridge of thyroid tissue that connects the left and right thyroid lobes.

Kelp: this is a 'health' product derived from seaweed and contains much iodine.

Lymph gland (lymph node): small glands that 'filter' lymph and when enlarged are most easily felt in the neck, under the arms, or in the groin.

Lymphadenoid goitre: the same as Hashimoto's goitre.

Lymphocyte: a particular type of white corpuscle that is concerned with the recognition of foreign proteins and the manufacture of antibodies.

Lymphoma: a malignant tumour of the lymphocytes that may involve the thyroid gland.

Medullary-cell cancer: a cancer of the medullary, C- or parafollicular cells that lodge in the thyroid gland and secrete the hormone calcitonin.

Metastases: a secondary deposit of cancer cells at a site distant to the original or primary cancer.

Methimazole: an antithyroid drug.

Microsomal antibodies: various techniques of increasing sensitivity (precipitin, latex, tanned red cells agglutination, enzyme-linked immunosorbent tests) are used to identify and quantify these antibodies. Microsomal antibodies are cytotoxic which means that they act against the thyroid cells and may destroy them.

They are present in most cases of Hashimoto's thyroiditis and some cases of Graves' disease.

Multinodular goitre: a goitre that contains many nodules. If you have a multinodular goitre you may be euthyroid now but you may later develop thyrotoxicosis.

Myxoedema: a severe advanced form of hypothyroidism. The term strictly applies to the thickened skin which is characteristic of severe hypothyroidism.

Neonatal: the first 4 weeks of a baby's life.

Neutrophil: a white corpuscle that very rarely is reduced in numbers as a side-effect of antithyroid drug treatment (see agranulocytosis).

Nodule: a lump in the thyroid gland.

Oculomotor muscles: these muscles control the movements of your eyeballs. They may become affected in Graves' ophthalmopathy.

Oestrogens: female ovarian hormones. Among their many other actions they increase the level of the thyroxine-binding proteins that carry thyroxine and T_3 in your bloodstream. When increased as in pregnancy or if you are taking an oestrogen-containing oral contraceptive 'pill', they cause elevation of the total but not the free thyroid hormones.

Ophthalmopathy: this comprises a variety of changes in the eyes that occur characteristically in some patients with Graves' disease.

Ophthalmoplegia: this is used to describe weakness or paralysis of the oculomotor muscles that move the eyeballs. Ophthalmoplegia may cause double vision (diplopia).

Orbit: the rigid bony socket in which the eye lies.

Osteoporosis: a thinning of the bones that occurs in women particularly at the time of the menopause and in men as they grow older. It is aggravated by hyperthyroidism.

Parathyroid glands: four little glands close to the thyroid that secrete the parathyroid hormone which controls the level of calcium in your blood.

Pernicious anaemia: see Addisonian anaemia. Pernicious is not a good word because the condition is easily treated.

Phaeochromocytoma: a tumour of the adrenal gland(s) that secretes hormones that affect your blood pressure.

Pituitary gland: an endocrine gland in the base of the skull that secretes a large number of different hormones. Of particular interest in thyroid disorders is the thyroid-stimulating hormone (TSH), also known as thyrotrophin.

Plummer's disease: named after the American physician who described it, is another name for a toxic multinodular goitre.

Postpartum: after labour.

Pretibial myxoedema: a skin condition usually affecting the lower legs and associated with Graves' disease in some patients. The term is misleading because it has nothing to do with *hypo*thyroidism.

Propylthiouracil: an antithyroid drug.

Proptosis: protrusion of the eyes. The same as exophthalmos.

Radio-iodine: there are three different radioactive isotopes of iodine which are used in the diagnosis of thyroid disorders. One isotope, I^{131}, is also used for the treatment of hyperthyroidism and thyroid cancer. The isotopes with a shorter duration of action (half-life), ^{123}I and ^{132}I, are often used for diagnostic tests.

Recurrent laryngeal nerves: these are the two nerves that supply the vocal cords. They may be injured during thyroid surgery and this causes huskiness of the voice.

Reflexes: the tendon reflexes, tested by your doctor tapping for example the tendon just below your knee-cap, may be slow to relax in hypothyroidism and unusually brisk in hyperthyroidism.

Replacement therapy: this is the use of a hormone given by your doctor to make good the deficient secretion by one of your endocrine glands.

Riedel's thyroiditis: a very rare form of hardening of the thyroid gland.

Scan: an examination by X-rays (CAT- or CT-scan), ultrasound (echo- or sono-gram) or radioisotopes (scintigram) which produces what amounts to three dimensional pictures of the organ being studied.

Sheehan's syndrome: hypopituitarism as a result of a postpartum haemorrhage. Hypothyroidism is one component of the resulting hormone deficiencies.

Sick euthyroid syndrome: this is a situation in which the patient is suffering from some severe non-thyroid illness in which the blood T_3 level is depressed, and also sometimes the T_4 level. In fact the patient is euthyroid and the TSH level is not raised. As recovery takes place the thyroid function tests return to normal.

Silent thyroiditis: an episode of hyperthyroidism due to an auto-immune disorder or perhaps sometimes to virus thyroiditis unaccompanied by any pain or discomfort in the thyroid gland. It is important that this is distinguished from Graves' disease by an isotope scan because the treatment is so different.

Stridor: a crowing noise made on breathing, usually when asleep, due to compression or displacement of the windpipe by a goitre.

Subacute viral thyroiditis: this is the same as viral thyroiditis or de Quervain's disease.

Suppurative thyroiditis: an acute infection of the thyroid gland by pus-making micro-organisms.

T_3 *toxicosis*: a state of hyperthyroidism caused by increased secretion of tri-iodothyronine unassociated with an increased blood level of T_4. The TSH level is suppressed. It may occur early in the course of Graves' disease.

Tetany: a condition due to a low calcium level in your blood that causes the muscles of your hands (and sometimes your feet) to go into spasm. It may occur from damage to the parathyroid glands during thyroid surgery.

Thymus: a gland in the upper chest behind the breast-bone that makes certain white corpuscles.

Thyroglobulin: a protein to which the thyroid hormones are attached when they are stored in the thyroid gland. Measurement of the blood level of thyroglobulin is valuable for telling that no normal or malignant thyroid cells are left after total removal of the thyroid gland and/or an ablative therapeutic dose of radio-iodine is given for the treatment of thyroid cancer. This test is also used for detecting if any metastases have developed.

Thyroglobulin antibodies: thyroglobulin antibodies are mainly directed against the thyroglobulin stored in the thyroid gland. Increased amounts are usually found in patients with Hashimoto's disease but the microsomal antibodies are usually more sensitive in establishing the diagnosis.

Thyroglossal duct: this is a remnant left behind as the thyroid gland descends from its origin at the base of the tongue to the neck in the unborn baby. It may become the site of a thyroglossal cyst.

Thyroid crisis or storm: an acute exacerbation of thyrotoxicosis that may be fatal unless treated promptly.

Thyroidectomy: this is the technical word for surgical removal of the thyroid gland. The surgeon may remove all of the gland (total thyroidectomy), the majority such as seven-eighths (subtotal thyroidectomy), or only a lobe (thyroid lobectomy).

Thyroiditis: this is an inflammatory condition of the thyroid gland that is usually caused by an auto-immune process (Hashimoto's thyroiditis) or by a virus (subacute viral or de Quervain's thyroiditis). There are other rarer forms of thyroiditis (see also 'silent thyroiditis').

Thyroid-stimulating antibodies: these antibodies, also known as thyrotrophin-receptor stimulating antibodies, occupy the TSH-receptor sites on the surface of thyroid cells and stimulate the cells to increase their secretion of thyroid hormones. They are probably the cause of auto-immune hyperthyroidism (Graves' disease). These thyroid-stimulating immunoglobulins can be detected in more than 90 per cent of such patients and also occur in 60 per cent of euthyroid patients who have ophthalmic Graves' disease. The same antibody occurs temporarily in some patients with Hashimoto's disease who may have a transient episode of hyperthyroidism ('Hashitoxicosis').

Thyroid-stimulating hormone (TSH): this is the hormone secreted by the pituitary gland that regulates the hormonal output from the thyroid gland. Its measurement is used to confirm the diagnosis of hypothyroidism (raised TSH level) and of hyperthyroidism (depressed TSH level). A low TSH level may also occur under a number of other circumstances:

- during the first 3 months of pregnancy in normal women;
- in some patients with eye symptoms indicative of Graves' ophthalmopathy before hyperthyroidism develops, and in those in whom hyperthyroidism never develops (ophthalmic Graves' disease);
- in patients who are in remission from, or have been cured, of Graves' disease. This happens because recovery of the previously suppressed pituitary is often delayed for many months;
- in patients with failure of the pituitary gland; and
- in any patient, but particularly the elderly, the secretion of TSH may be reduced by non-thyroidal illnesses either physical or psychiatric.

Thyrotrophin-releasing hormone (TRH): this hormone is secreted by the hypothalamus and increases the activity of the cells in the pituitary that secrete thyroid-stimulating hormone (TSH).

Thyrotrophin-releasing hormone (TRH) test: this test is seldom used now that there is a sensitive TSH assay that reliably measures reduced levels of the thyroid-stimulating hormone.

Thyrotoxicosis: another name for hyperthyroidism or thyroid overactivity.

Thyroxine: one of the thyroid hormones, which contains four iodine atoms and is often called T_4.

Thyroxine-binding globulin (TBG): three main classes of protein carry thyroxine in the bloodstream—globulin, pre-albumin, and albumin. The most important of these is globulin which carries about 70 per cent of the thyroxine. In some laboratories the TBG is measured as an alternative to, or as an additional check on, the T_3-resin-binding test. An abnormally low, even absent, or an abnormally high level of thyroxine-binding globulin level may occur as an innocent hereditary abnormality, usually in men. When the TBG is low, the levels of total T_4 and total T_3 are also low, because the main carrier-protein is reduced; when the TBG is high, the level of the thyroid hormones is raised, but in both situations the patient is euthyroid and has a normal TSH level and usually a normal free T_4 and a normal free T_3.

Total serum thyroxine (T_4) level: this test, which is done on a small sample of blood removed from a vein, measures the total amount of thyroxine per unit of blood and this comprises the T_4 bound to the various different proteins which carry most of the thyroxine. The result may be expressed in terms of the weight of thyroxine per 100 ml of blood (micrograms/100 ml or $\mu g/100$ ml) or in terms of the number of molecules of thyroxine per litre (nanomoles/L or nmol/L). The normal reference ranges may differ slightly from one laboratory to another depending on the exact chemicals (reagents) used and the population of 'healthy' people from whose results the normal range has been derived. In most instances of hyperthyroidism, except of course T_3-toxicosis, the result of the T_4 estimation is unequivocally raised, and in patients with hypothyroidism it is reduced.

The main snag about measuring the total serum T_4 level is that the result depends on the amount of thyroxine bound to the carrier-proteins. It is the tiny amount of thyroxine which is unbound and floating free in the water of the blood that determines your thyroid status. Thus the result of the total thyroxine assay is influenced by two factors—the amount of T_4 present and the amount, and the binding capacity of the different carrier-proteins.

Under certain circumstances, for example in pregnancy, if you are taking the contraceptive pill containing oestrogens or you are having hormone replacement therapy (HRT) during the menopause, the amount of carrier-proteins is increased. This increases the total T_4 level but does not make you hyperthyroid because the free non-protein-bound thyroxine remains normal. Certain drugs, such as aspirin and many others, may occupy the binding sites on the carrier-proteins normally reserved for thyroxine. These drugs will therefore tend to lower the total T_4 level by displacing the protein-bound thyroxine.

Because variations in the amount of the carrier-proteins and in the number of their binding sites may be induced by hormones, drugs, many non-thyroid diseases and by genetic factors, various additional tests are often done to make appropriate allowance for these changes (see T_3-resin uptake test).

Total serum triiodothyronine (T_3) level: this measure of the total serum protein-bound concentration of T_3 has the same disadvantages as measuring the total serum T_4 level. Usually the total T_3 and T_4 levels move in parallel because about one-third of the T_3 is secreted by the thyroid gland and two-thirds is derived in peripheral tissues from the conversion of T_4 to T_3. In T_3-toxicosis the total T_3 is raised but the total T_4 is normal; similarly the free T_3 is usually raised and the free T_4 is normal. In hypothyroidism the T_3 level is often less depressed than the T_4 level which is a better indicator of thyroid deficiency but the TSH level is an even more sensitive test.

Trachea: the windpipe, which may be compressed or displaced by a goitre.

Triiodothyronine: colloquially known as T_3 is one of the two thyroid hormones.

Triiodothyronine (T$_3$)-resin-binding test: this is used to make allowance for variations in the binding proteins. There can, however, be few tests which, because of its name, has caused more confusion among patients and also among their doctors than this one! It is in essence a procedure designed to determine how much a high or a low total thyroxine level is the consequence of changes in the amount of carrier-proteins or in the available sites on these proteins for binding thyroxine molecules. The technique is *not* in any way a measure of the total or free triiodothyronine level.

By itself the T_3-resin-binding test is of little value; it is used to 'correct' the value of the total serum thyroxine, and this correction is incorporated in the 'free thyroxine index'.

Tumour: a tumour is a lump or nodule that in the context of this book can be felt in the thyroid gland. It may be benign or cancerous.

Ultra-sound: this is a technique for determining the structure of an organ. It is useful for investigating a goitre and may reveal a nodule or nodules that cannot be felt by your doctor, and show whether the lump is solid or cystic (filled with fluid).

Vitamin B$_{12}$: failure to absorb this vitamin causes Addisonian anaemia. This is an auto-immune disorder caused by the destruction of certain cells in the stomach wall that secrete the intrinsic factor that facilitates the absorption of vitamin B$_{12}$. Addisonian anaemia may occur as an accompaniment of thyroid auto-immune disease.

Vitiligo: this is a skin condition characterized by patches of depigmentation sometimes surrounded by a thin rim of hyperpigmentation. It is an auto-immune disorder that may act as a marker for other auto-immune disorders.

Viral thyroiditis: this is the same as subacute viral thyroiditis or de Quervain's disease.

Von Basedow's disease: this is the same as Graves' disease and named after the German doctor who also described the disease. It is the name used on the continent of Europe for diffuse toxic goitre.

Glossary of drugs

Throughout the text the 'common' name has been used for each drug mentioned, names likely to be familiar to doctors world-wide. Doctors sometimes prescribe drugs of a particular proprietary brand and this may confuse the patient who may not know the chemical content of the proprietary tablet.

Below is a short glossary of the drugs most often used in the treatment of patients with thyroid disorders. In each instance the drug is identified first by its common name and then by its official name as it appears in the pharmacopoeia. This is followed by a list of proprietary names, a list that cannot be all-inclusive because different brand names are used in different countries and in different marketing areas throughout the world. Finally a brief indication is given of the purpose for which the drug is usually used.

Thyroxine (T₄)

Official names: levothyroxine sodium, L-thyroxine sodium, levothyroxinum natricum, thyroxine sodium.

Proprietary names: Cytoden, Cytolen, Eltroxin, Euthyrox, Letter, Levaxin, Levoid, Levothroid, Levothyronin, Oroxine, Percutacrine, Synthroid, Thyratabs, Thyrine, Thyro-4, Thyrohormone, Thyroxevan, Thyroxinal, Thyroxinique, Trio-4.

Use: as replacement therapy in deficiency of thyroid hormone; for treatment of goitre.

Triiodothyronine (T₃)

Official names: liothyronine sodium, liothyroninum natricum, L-tri-iodothyronine, sodium liothyronine, triiodothyronine sodium.

Proprietary names: Cynomel, Cytomel, Tertroxin, Triacana, Trithyrone.

Use: as replacement therapy in deficiency of thyroid hormones.

Mixtures of thyroxine and triiodothyronine

Official names: none.

Proprietary names: Liotrix (available in a range of strengths containing T_4 and T_3 in a 4:1 ratio), Dithyron (thyroxine 0.05 mg and triiodothyronine 12.5 μg), Euthroid, Thyrolar (thyroxine 0.05 mg and triiodothyronine 12.5 μg).

Use: as replacement therapy in deficiency of thyroid hormones but have no advantage over thyroxine alone.

Thyroglobulin

Official name: thyroglobulin.

Proprietary name: Proloid.

Use: as replacement therapy in deficiency of thyroid hormones but seldom used nowadays and has no advantage over thyroxine.

Thyroid extract

Official names: dry thyroid, Getrocknete Schilddruse, thyroid extract, thyreoidin, thyroidea, thyroideum sicca, tiroide secca.

Proprietary names: S-P-T, Thyranon, Thyrar, Thyroboline, Thyrocine.

Use: as replacement therapy in deficiency of thyroid hormone, but has now been superseded by thyroxine because thyroid extract is not a pure substance.

Carbimazole

Official names: carbimazole, carbimazolum.

Proprietary names: Carbazole, Neo-mercazole, Neo-morphazole, Neo-thyreostat, Thyrostat.

Use: for control or treatment of thyroid overactivity.

Methimazole

Official names: methimazole, mercazolylum, thiamazolum.

Proprietary names: Favistan, Tapazole, Thacapzol.

Use: for control or treatment of thyroid overactivity.

Propylthiouracil

Official names: propylthiouracil, propylthiouracilum.

Proprietary names: Propycil, Propyl-thyracil, Thyreostat II, Tiotil.

Use: for control or treatment of thyroid overactivity.

Propranolol

Official names: propranolol, propranolol hydrochloride.

Proprietary names: Aviocardyl, Berkolol, Dociton, Herzul, Inderal, Inderalici, Kemi, Sumial.

Use: to slow the heart rate and reduce other symptoms of thyroid overactivity.

Index